Medical Adventures in the Arctic

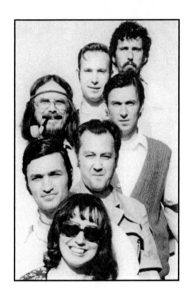

including the true story of
Canada's Impostor Surgeon

by

Lianne Lacroix, MD

Webb Publishing
Kelowna, BC

Illustrations by Lianne Lacroix
Editing, book design and cover design by Jill Veitch & Barb Sutherland, Webb Publishing.ca
Author photo by Glenn Durrell Photography
Photo and credit on last page translated from San Sebastian Clinic website.

Library and Archives Canada Cataloguing in Publication

Lacroix, Lianne, 1943-
    Medical adventures in the Arctic : including the true story of Canada's impostor surgeon / by Lianne Lacroix.

ISBN 978-0-9812945-3-7

    1. Lacroix, Lianne, 1943-. 2. Women physicians--Northwest Territories--Inuvik--Biography. 3. DiStefano, Angelo. 4. Surgeons--Northwest Territories--Inuvik--Biography. 5. Inuvik (N.W.T.)--Biography. I. Title.

R464.L33A3 2010   610.92   C2010-901765-X

Printed in Canada

Table of Contents

Preface

It was a quiet Saturday morning, unusual for the busy regional hospital. After making rounds I sat down at a table in the nurse's station and began an engaging conversation with a new doctor in town. We discovered that we had both worked in Inuvik, Northwest Territories, in the Canadian Arctic. I had spent the first four years of my professional career there in the 1970's, some thirty years ago, and he spent a few months there every summer doing vacation relief for doctors on holidays.

"Were you there at the same time as that impostor surgeon?" he asked.

Surprised, I answered, "Why yes I was, but he was not an impostor, even if the newspapers called him one! He was a highly trained surgeon who got caught in a love triangle."

"Must be quite a story," he said

I felt a shot of energy. "I should write a book!" I exclaimed.

It dawned on me in that moment that I must record the story of Dr. Angelo DiStefano for all to read. I was there, and I know what really happened. I could not let my friend's reputation sour into the legend of a scoundrel, especially since the truth was so much more interesting.

But memories of the arctic were far away in my mind. It had been thirty years since my northern adventures. My medical practice was always so busy, and family life seemed to occupy the rest of my time.

Lianne Lacroix

Several months after my conversation with the new doctor, my husband and I began to de-clutter our house. In the back of the garage sat an old trunk full of arctic mementos: Eskimo carvings, moth-eaten furs and assorted papers.

In one large brown envelope I discovered three postcards and ten letters in Angelo DiStefano's wispy handwriting. His strong Italian accent and lively voice came back to me and memories flooded into my mind. Though he was with us for only a year and a half before he was escorted out of the country, he had made a big impression on our small-knit community of physicians, personally and professionally.

The time was right to record the memories of my unique and wonderful experience in the arctic in the mid-1970's, and to clear the air about our 'impostor surgeon'. While day to day events all blend together in my mind, and many names and faces are forgotten, the medical emergencies and extraordinary moments remain crystal clear. I was the lone female in a group of keen and lively young doctors; we were learning our profession and enjoying a once in a lifetime experience in the northernmost region of Canada.

ONE

The Arctic Beckons

It all started in the summer of 1973. I was sitting in a plane, a PWA (Pacific Western Airlines) Boeing 737 at 30,000 feet, flying away from my home in Ottawa to start a new job in Inuvik, Northwest Territories. Inuvik is beyond the Arctic Circle, and besides that, I did not know much else about the place. I was a little tense, unaware of the adventures and difficulties in store as I was about to start my first fulltime job as a medical doctor.

I graduated from Ottawa Medical School in 1972 and then finished a twelve month rotating internship at the Ottawa Civic Hospital. At 30 years old, I was a slim, dark haired, greenish-brown-eyed woman from a French Canadian Ottawa Valley family, who was looking at the next chapter of her life.

I left my life in Ottawa because I knew my time was up; I must leave. I did not want to set up a practice locally or join another doctor in the small town where I had grown up. It did not feel right. I felt sure that my life was somewhere else with a person whom I was yet to meet. I dared hope to find my life companion and get married within the next few years.

My best friend, Monique, had graduated with me the year before and said at the time, "I see you with a young man of German descent." How strange, I thought, yet I respected her uncanny sense of intuition that so often proved correct. After graduation, Monique had married our classmate Denis and moved to Montreal. My life was not to be in that fair city, either.

While I was in medical school I spent my summers in Quebec, working on the east coast of James Bay in a sub-arctic Cree Indian village called Fort George. I enjoyed the close-to-the-land lifestyle and the interesting people and thought perhaps my new life would start there. I enquired and found that Fort George had a permanent doctor and no job for me. I was relieved in a way. My closest summer friends had all moved somewhere else and I knew that I would not resurrect those happy moments again.

The summer of 1973 was a strange period of pause in my life. I spent much of it waiting and waiting to hear if I had been accepted for a job in Northern Medical Services through Health and Welfare Canada. I often sat on a lawn chair in the tiny yard of my parents' new house in Ottawa. They had sold the farm and moved to town where my father continued work as a construction inspector. Finally after almost two months I received a letter saying that I was hired and should report to the hospital at Inuvik, Northwest Territories. I grabbed a map of Canada and searched for Inuvik, finding it 3000 miles from Ottawa on the northernmost edge of the North American continent, along the arctic Beaufort Sea.

I felt a bit scared, but was excited at the prospect of new adventures. Although a very careful and mild person, I knew this journey would appeal to my bold and determined side. I packed my bags and left. The trip would take two days by plane with an overnight stop at an Edmonton hotel. The second day of travel included stops at Hay River and Norman Wells, and a further five hours to Inuvik. As I headed higher and deeper north, I had a great deal of time to reflect on my journey thus far.

I grew up on a farm twenty-five miles southeast of Ottawa, the eldest of six children. I always dreamed of a post-secondary education, but as I grew into my teens, I knew that my family could not afford to help me financially. I didn't realize at the time how lucky I was that my father was able to support his children without obliging me to find menial jobs to help out. Even though I was the eldest child, he gave me the greatest gift of all, the gift of *freedom* to plan the course of my own life. It took me many years to understand how precious this gift was, as I later saw several young women of my generation limited by their commitment to family.

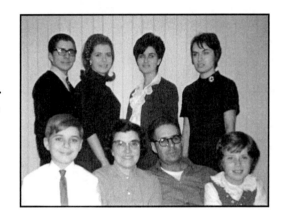

**Farm family, circa 1965.
Back: Philip, Christine,
Rachel, Lianne.
Front: Maurice, my
mother-Laurence, my
father-Leonard,
Francine.**

After I graduated at the top of my small high school class, I travelled to Ottawa and took one year of university, called grade 13, so that I would qualify to be accepted into the laboratory technologist program at Ottawa General Hospital. We apprenticed and worked at the hospital during this 18 month program and were paid the tiny wage of $100 per month. This was just enough to cover room and board at a residence for young women run by an order of nuns.

At this point it might be expected that I would reveal my dislike of the strict residence rules and recount my escapades to defy them, but such was not my case. I loved the order, the cleanliness and the rules of curfew that seemed totally reasonable to me.

I knew that the lab tech course was a stepping stone toward the true work of my life; neither did I want to marry a farmer next door and raise a family. It just did not feel right to me. Even though I had no money, I wanted something different from my life. Perhaps I would do research like Madame Curie or work in a country far away in the missions like my aunt, who was a missionary nun in Papua New Guinea. I had read the story of Africa's Dr. Sweitzer in our high school's sparse library. I would find something interesting. I did not, however, feel called to become a nun.

Plus, I was convinced that I would find the right man for me, somewhere. After finishing my lab tech course I spent the required year working at the hospital, wondering what to do next.

Then one day as I worked in Biochemistry collecting blood samples from patients and performing the manual chemistry tests, I took a late lunch in the cafeteria. It was a winter day and the bright cold rays of sunlight gleamed on the shiny waxed floor.

Just then in a moment of blinding clarity, I saw my future in front of my eyes like a vision; a veil was lifted for a moment. The path was clear and I knew at that one instant that I must become a doctor.

It seemed an impossible dream to me. I had no money, and it took so long, seven years I was told. Yet my heart was filled with joy for the road was finally clear. I told no one about this idea for several months. The only doctor that I knew was my childhood doctor, but my good health had prevented more than one or two visits.

I wrote to the Ottawa University and asked for their curriculum booklet and read it over and over. "Hmm, perhaps I could take those courses; they do seem interesting," I thought. Being a practical person, I went to the psychology department at Ottawa U and requested that they perform some intelligence tests to see if I could *make* it. After a day of tests they said that my visual memory was very good but my math was not strong. "No problem," I thought, "I will count pills very carefully." Then I told my family about my dream. They were surprised, but quite supportive.

I could not apply for student loans since I was no longer a student. There was only one solution. I must work one more year while saving enough money for my first year of pre-med. Then I would be a student and could apply for the bursary-loans. I had arrived at one of those life altering moments where two roads diverge and the one chosen makes all the difference.

Lab Tech Days: Fort George, 1964

For the two years that I worked as a lab tech before starting my new studies at Ottawa U. I joined a Christian youth group called Mundo. We met once a month to encourage young people to work in third world countries and to raise money to send medical supplies. We often invited speakers to tell us about their work and to recruit for various countries.

Somehow I was never attracted to hot countries, likely because my ancestors had lived so long in northern countries that my genes had adapted to the cold. One day as I worked in the hospital lab, a nurse that I had met at Mundo called to offer me a job in Fort George, Quebec, where I would be setting up a laboratory in a thirty bed hospital.

I jumped at this chance and headed to the Cree village of 1300 people. It was situated on an island along a beautiful large river that empties into the eastern side of James Bay. My experience there was a wonderful fantastic period of deep friendships, fascinating native people unspoiled in their way of life and magnificent rivers and woods where we fished, camped and even hunted with local guides.

I remember well the first day that I landed on the river at Fort George aboard a Canso amphibian airplane after travelling by train for three days from Ottawa. It was my first experience on an airplane and although rather scared, I was amazed at the views of the country from the air and quite enjoyed the experience. This July day, the sun was shining on a golden sandy beach along the shore with hundreds of laughing native people standing on the banks waiting for the plane to arrive. The plane passengers boarded a large canoe powered by an outboard motor as we made our way to shore.

Tall evergreens covered part of the background with many small houses and several tepees along the road to town. As I stepped ashore a great positive feeling came over me and I felt that I was entering a golden adventure and something very special.

The hospital of Fort George was managed by an order of nuns at the Catholic Mission. The nurse in charge, energetic cheerful Sister Gisele, has remained a friend some forty years later. The hospital contained 30 beds with one doctor, a dozen registered and practical nurses, and one laboratory technologist: me. I set up the lab in a tiny ten feet by six feet room that had a large window. I soon became close friends with Lucille and Rita, who were nurse practitioners before that word was ever invented. They both worked in the outpatient clinic room where patients just showed up for medical care without appointments. There were no phones. The nurses saw all the patients, treated them and triaged them for the doctor who saw only the seriously ill.

We all worked from 8 am until noon then took two hours off during the slower period of the day and worked again until 6 or 7 pm. In the evening I would accompany Lucille to visit sick and elderly people in the village. She spoke fairly good Cree and I listened and learned some Cree Indian words as well.

There was no alcohol available in the village so police were not necessary; there were very few crimes. It was a close knit community where the people lived close to the land, trapping, hunting and fishing.

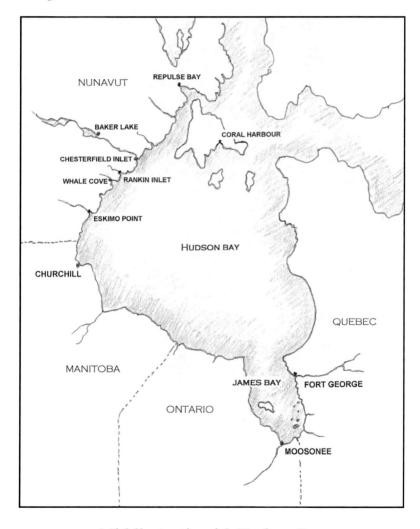

Middle Arctic with Hudson Bay

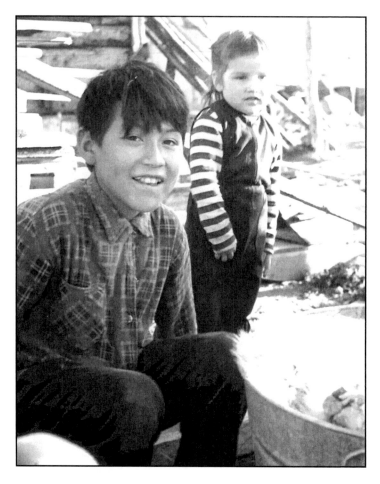

Fort George children, circa 1965.

Skidoos were not yet in common use. People kept large teams of fierce Huskies that were working dogs and not pets. We treated dog bites fairly often at the hospital.

In the winter, when we weren't working, the hospital staff explored the several miles of scenery across the island on some early skidoos (two person snowmobiles). In the summer we went camping and fishing by large canoe, employing local native guides. It was an isolated world of its own with no TV or radio and our only contact with the rest of the world was the mail carried twice weekly by bush plane and the Mission's two way radio.

After thirteen months of working in my small laboratory I returned to Ottawa and started my first year of pre-med BA at the University of Ottawa. I was fortunate to be able to return to sub-arctic Fort George every summer for five more years to work as lab tech from May through August and save money for my university years.

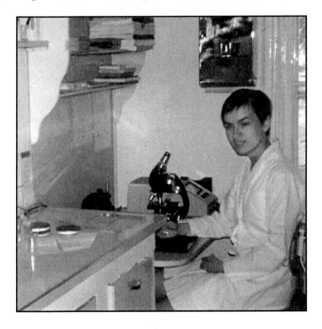

Lab tech of Fort George, 1965.

During those northern summers, our special treat was a picnic on the Brothers' boat, a 60 foot diesel powered schooner that transported provisions between Moosonee and Fort George during the summer.

The captain was a cheerful 45 year old Oblate Brother who spoke Cree and was fond of story telling.

The picnic was an annual but informal event. About twenty people from the Mission and hospital would spend most of the day on the boat. We would putt along the large river enjoying lunch on board and then travel into James Bay close to shore. We admired the evergreen forested lands and the great expanse of bright blue sky while rolling along the salty waves of the inland sea. When the orange and mauve sunset glowed in the evening sky, we would return to our dock feeling rested deep in our hearts.

At the end of one summer, just as the time came for me to return to Ottawa, I had the fantastic opportunity of spending three days travelling south to Moosonee with the Brother and his three Cree speaking crewmen. We left early one cloudy windy morning, just me and the men. I sat on deck that day wearing my raincoat and rubber boots, rolling in time with the boat as it crested the choppy waters of the large inland water. Keeping my eyes fixed on the horizon prevented any sea sickness. The native pilot guided our way along not far from shore, nicely avoiding the sandbars and rocks. As evening came the strong winds calmed down and we anchored in a sheltered bay overnight.

The brother prayed and slept in a tiny cabin on deck beside the wheelhouse while the crew slept in bunks in the spotlessly clean engine room. I slept in a sleeping bag resting on a mattress thrown over barrels in the hold near the small kitchen. "Make sure you don't fall overboard during the night," said the Brother to me as he wished me goodnight.

We were far away from any settlement. None of us could swim to shore in the icy waters; native people never swam in northern rivers. It was very dark and as I made my way to the hold I gazed at the sky in wonder. Never had I seen a sky so dark with stars so bright, it was like a great velvet dome pierced by millions of diamond stars.

The next day we continued our journey until mid-afternoon when we stopped on an uninhabited island in the middle of James Bay to go duck hunting. We walked along the deep wet grasses bordering a stream. The crew members shot a couple of ducks and missed another. Then the Brother handed me his shot gun and said quietly, "There's a duck over there. You shoot it."

He and I had practiced target shooting before, and he knew that I was a good shot. I aimed and fired, and the duck fell! I had shot my first duck. It impressed the crewmen, but I felt so terrible that I promised myself I would never kill another creature higher than fish on the evolutionary scale. The ducks were cooked in our small wood stove and eaten by all.

Here I was, a young woman alone with four men on an uninhabited island in the middle of a great northern sea. I felt totally safe and trusted the Brother's friendship implicitly. Perhaps he was a father figure for me and I aimed to please him by fitting into northern life and belonging to the magnificent land. I was not a tourist and I was keenly aware that this was a wonderful unique experience that was a rare and precious gift to me.

After one more day of chugging along in good weather, we docked in Moosonee by late afternoon. There was nobody to greet us but we managed to find a man with a truck to give us a ride to the Mission building. The native crew walked over to houses of their relatives. The next day, I said goodbye to the Brother. I shook his hand but gratitude choked my words - we did not hug in the sixties except with very close family members.

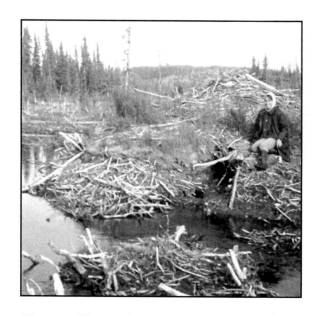

Abandoned beaver dam on an island, mid-James Bay.

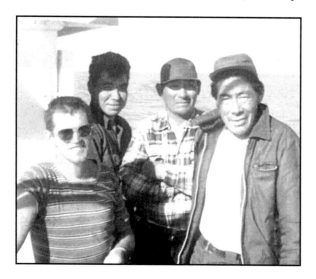

The Brother (left) and crew of the schooner.

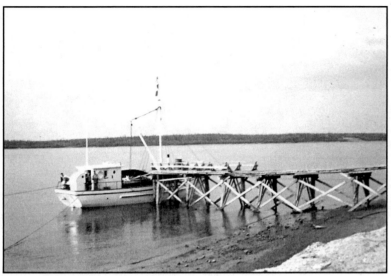

The Brother's schooner, unloading supplies at low tide.

I took a plane back to Ottawa and continued my studies, feeling that I had returned from a far away world.

While in medical school, I stayed with my parents, paying a small amount of rent to help with the household that still held the three youngest children. I enjoyed medical school and made several very good friends. I never returned to Fort George after I graduated, but those years have never left my soul. I still dream about walking along the golden beaches, following the movements of the tides and admiring the glowing sunsets. It was a time spent wondering about my future.

These were the memories that filled my thoughts as I looked out the window across thinning evergreen forests pock-marked by thousands of shallow lakes, until we finally started to descend into Inuvik.

Lianne Lacroix

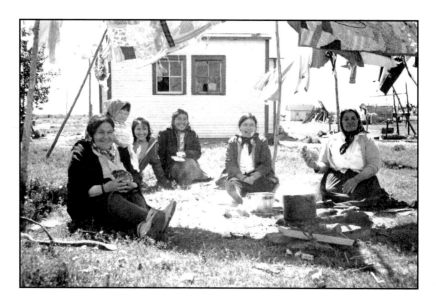

The people of Fort George.

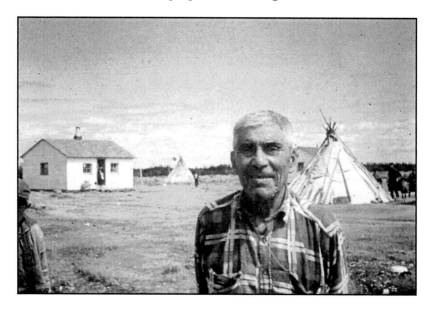

TWO

Midnight Sun: 1973

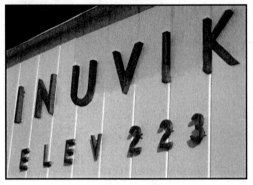

The flight had been very smooth and the weather remained stable and warm at 75°F on a late afternoon in July.

I looked at my fellow passengers. Most of them were casually dressed young men wearing plain blue jeans and checkered shirts sporting beards or moustaches. I felt a little out of place in my French blue suit and platform shoes that were the latest style in 1973. My fashion was but a thin veneer on a farm girl who would soon feel at home in the untamed land.

There are many reasons people travel to the arctic. The summer brought geologists looking for gold or natural gas, researchers and university students studying everything from the migration of caribou (arctic deer) to the seasons of arctic mice. There were teachers, RCMP officers, armed forces personnel, pilots and hospital personnel, plus trappers and local native Dene Indians and Inuit people. I remember thinking that this would actually be a very good place to meet an interesting life companion.

The large plane touched down gently. From the windows, rows of scraggly evergreen trees covered the flat terrain, but there was no sign of civilization. No buildings were visible until the plane turned and the airport building appeared. It was a plain low structure, painted blue, topped by a squat control tower. The large room inside was filled with noisy people trying to retrieve their bags from a simple cart.

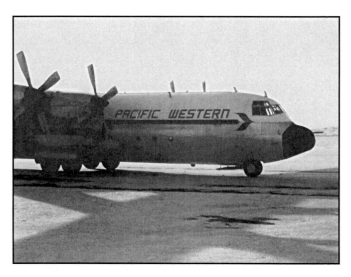

A PWA freight plane typical of the day.

I knew that the hospital would likely send somebody to meet me, so I was not overly concerned in this room filled with strangers. As I found my bags, a voice behind me said; "Are you the new doctor for the hospital?" I turned around and faced a man around my own age with shoulder length copper coloured hair held by a fur headband on his forehead.

"Hi. Bill Sara," he said, extending a firm handshake.

"Hi," I said as I introduced myself.

He grabbed my largest bag, I grabbed the small one and we walked to a large green station wagon with the Northern Health logo on the door. A large white dog that looked like an albino German shepherd sat on the back seat. I hesitated.

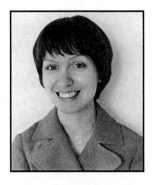

New doctor in town.

"This is Gus," Bill said reassuringly.

We drove in silence for a few minutes, down a gravel road bordered on both sides by spindly evergreens.

"How far is the town?" I asked

"Not far, about seven or eight miles," he answered.

Then silence again. He was not the chatty type but I did not get a bad feeling from him.

When meeting a new person, especially a man, I am always careful, concerned for my safety. Perhaps it is an instinct of survival for a young woman and it had served me well so far in my life.

We drove along in silence for a few more minutes until my curiosity was awakened. He must be a hospital worker, I thought, maybe an orderly or a handy man. In the arctic a small hospital might send any available worker to meet a new doctor.

Finally I asked, "What kind of work do you do at the hospital?"

An amused look crossed his face. "I'm the Chief of staff," he answered, which meant that he was the senior doctor!

I relaxed and allowed my first shy smile. "A colleague," I thought! Wonderful, I could relate to any kind of doctor after seven years of medical school. I felt suddenly reassured, and even warm in my heart. He was a colleague, perhaps a friend. My new life was beginning and I was just meeting the first character in this new adventure.

We drove around a low hill and past the dark brown hospital building to the hospital guest house where I would stay until being assigned an apartment. Several wooden pastel-coloured houses could be seen along the unpaved street as the sun was going down in the western sky.

"See you tomorrow at 8 am," said Bill curtly as he drove off. Another reserved character. Like me, I thought.

After unpacking briefly, I sat in the plain but pleasant living room and watched the light from the sun just above the horizon where it circled, heading for the northern sky.

Happy cries of baseball players could be heard in the distance from local children and adults playing baseball all night. I was to learn that in the summer the native people follow no clock, eating and sleeping as nature dictates.

Finally at midnight I took a photo of the side of the pink clapboard house illuminated by the low sun shining directly from the north. I was looking at the famous midnight sun of legend. Yes, this land was different, unusual. Some would call it strange.

I went upstairs and found a bedroom. The windows were covered by kitchen aluminum foil to try to trick the body into sleep. Perhaps this exotic place will become my home I thought, as I drifted to sleep...

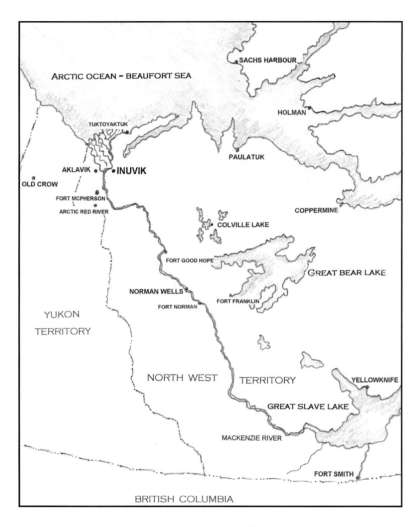

Western Arctic

Inuvik General Hospital: July 1973

The next morning I walked to the hospital and Bill showed me around. The doctors at Inuvik General Hospital were hired by Health and Welfare, a federal government department that looked after medical services for northern residents in the 1970's. We were salaried and paid around $18,000 per year. Our rent for furnished houses or apartments was deducted from that amount. This seemed fair to me at the time and I looked forward to paying back my $8,000 student debt within a year.

Usually the hospital employed four to five doctors and one surgeon to care for approximately 9000 people living within a 600 mile diameter of Inuvik: 4000 people lived in town and another 5000 people were spread across twelve villages. The region extended north 300 miles to Sachs Harbour, an Inuit settlement on Banks Island, and south 350 miles to Norman Wells and the Dene settlement of Fort Norman. Our western border was in the Yukon, 200 miles away at Old Crow, and our eastern border ran from Paulatuk, 300 miles northeast of us, to Fort Franklin, 300 miles in the southeast.

Inuvik was the central town. We had a 50 bed hospital and a nurses' residence close by where nurses could rent a room. Doctors rented a small assigned home, townhouse or apartment within walking distance to the hospital.

Many doctors came for one year or two, usually arriving or leaving in the summer. A few stayed much longer. Summer also brought locums: replacement doctors who stayed for a month or two while the permanent doctors went south for holidays or extra training. Two or three of the family doctors practiced anesthesia for surgeries.

For recreation the summer brought hiking, fishing, canoeing and exploration trips down rivers. Swimming was not possible as there were no beaches along the low lying delta of the Mackenzie River. There was an occasional water skier on the small lake behind the hospital.

We traveled a lot. Each doctor was assigned a village or two to visit every month. We always visited the same place, thus getting to know the people and developing a working rapport with the nurses. Any patient evacuated to our hospital from "my" village would automatically come under my care.

Every village had a nursing station where one to three nurse practitioners and midwives looked after the health needs of the native population. The northern communities were mostly Eskimo, now called Inuit, and the southern villages were native Indian people, now known as Dene. The nursing station carried various medications that were supplied free of charge to the population. There were no pharmacies.

Some nursing stations delivered low risk pregnancies and births, where the nurse was a midwife or had extra training in obstetrics and the mother had already given birth once. There were no roads and these villages could only be reached by airplanes.

Difficult cases were evacuated by med-evacs, as we called them. Patients were sent by plane to our hospital in Inuvik and then if necessary to our tertiary hospital in Edmonton, Alberta. A doctor or a nurse would accompany the patient on these trips.

Respiratory illnesses with pneumonia and sick children were the main illnesses in our patient population. We rarely saw heart problems or diabetes as the people still partially followed the traditional lifestyle and lived on the land and in fishing camps, hunting, fishing and walking constantly.

Every Thursday morning at 8 am we held an old fashioned Grand Rounds at the hospital, where all doctors met at one end of the hospital and reviewed the patients while walking from one room to another. Each doctor presented the patients under their care and discussed all aspects of their medical problems. This usually lasted until noon, then we all ate together in the boardroom near the cafeteria where we discussed patients and the medical workings and problems of the hospital.

Once a month, a specialist from Edmonton would come for several days to see patients that we had prepared for him. We never saw a female specialist in those days. The specialist would give us a medical lecture at noon on Thursdays and they also did special work for us. For example, an ENT (ears, nose and throat) surgeon repaired damaged eardrums in a dozen children during one weeklong trip. We saw numerous cases of ear infections with eardrum perforations, and it would have been difficult to send all these children to the hospital in Edmonton. We also found that the changes in altitude on their flight back to Inuvik often caused the eardrums to perforate again just after the repair.

The medical staff worked together very closely and shared easily in all the medical work. Our desks, which were all together in one common room, held a dictaphone so we dictated all our patient notes. Our medical secretary Corrine typed them for the patient files. Never had I seen such wonderfully legible and complete patient medical files. Even if doctor turnover was high, the file continued telling the complete medical story of each person that came to our hospital. Every few months we would award the "Golden Dictaphone" to the doctor who had fallen behind in doing his paperwork. It was an old dictaphone painted gold and I am proud to say that it never once graced my desk.

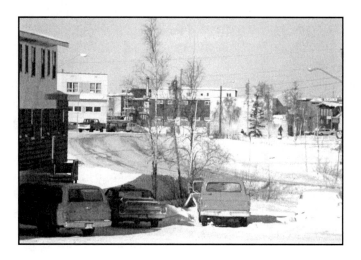

Inuvik

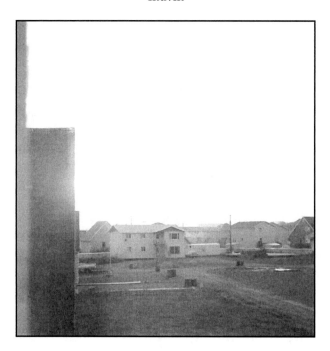

My first Midnight Sun.

First Surgeon: Summer 1973

When I first arrived in Inuvik in July 1973, the resident surgeon was an eccentric Frenchman from France, named Philippe. He was a short dark-eyed wiry man who was a true loner, never associating with any other staff and barely speaking to anyone.

"I'll try to speak with him since I speak his language," I said to Rob, the other young doctor who had just arrived in the summer. So I sat with Philippe in the hospital cafeteria one day and tried some polite conversation in French. No luck. He never looked at me once. His gaze was focused one foot to the left of my head and ten feet behind. I could not meet his eyes. He never smiled. It was very hard to have any conversation with him at all.

We had heard that he had worked in French Vietnam some years before. His surgical skills were dubious at best and he inspired little confidence in his colleagues. The doctors kept a close eye on his medical work so that no patient would be harmed.

On weekends he never visited anyone but went instead on long walks, alone, all day long, in the deep wilderness, with only a light backpack. We were surprised every time when he returned to his apartment. We would joke that surely he must be an android.

Decades later we would have identified him as a highly functioning autistic person with Asperger syndrome. That condition was not well known in medical circles at the time. Philippe did not stay in Inuvik very long and within a few months departed for places unknown.

Toga Party: Summer 1973

By the middle of August, I had become friends with a lovely nurse called Melodie, who lived in my apartment building. She was a second generation Canadian of Japanese ancestry, from British Columbia.

"I often get asked if I'm from the eastern arctic," Melodie told me. "The locals think I'm eastern arctic Eskimo!"

Certainly proves the theory of ancient migration from Asia across the Bering Strait, I thought.

One day we heard that the nurses had decided to hold a Roman toga party at the nurses' residence and we were all invited. However we would only be admitted if wearing the proper bed sheet toga.

The designated day arrived clear and hot with the evening sun circling around the sky. Coloured sheets were popular at the time and I spent a long time arranging my deep pink bed sheet around my body, over one shoulder and tightly held by several hidden safety pins. To me it looked like a good copy of a Hollywood-style Roman toga. I met Melodie at the door of our apartment building. She looked exotic in her light yellow bed sheet, I mean toga.

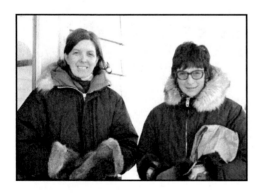

Two arctic nurse practitioners.

Lianne Lacroix

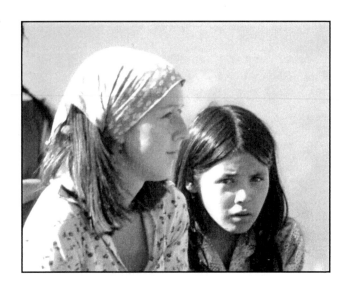

Two nurses attending hospital picnic.

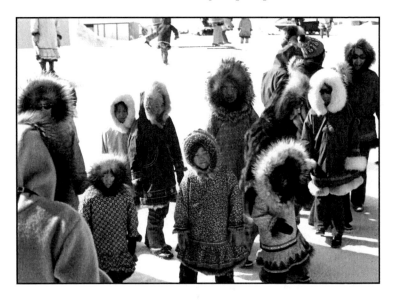

Kids in the arctic.

The nurses' residence had a large living room which had been emptied of all furniture except for cushions, and the windows were covered with foil to simulate darkness. It was decorated on a Roman theme with plastic flowers, spruce branches and bunches of real grapes taped to the walls. There were trays of cheese and crackers plus the grapes and many bottles of wine and beer. All eligible friends or acquaintances of the nurses had been invited. Music played from records and the dancing soon began. Most had bare feet or sandals and looked sufficiently exotic in their odd arrangements of multi-coloured bed sheets.

There was a young locum working at the hospital for a few weeks that summer. His name was Noah and he was of Inuit and European ancestry, from a prominent family in Sachs Harbour. This intrigued me since he was perhaps the first native person from the high arctic to make it through medical school. I had seen him in the hospital but not spoken to him. I was planning to congratulate him on his achievement of becoming a doctor against what I considered to be great odds.

I said hello and he asked me to dance in that 70's style where we stood two feet apart and moved our arms and feet to disco music. I introduced myself and told him that I was a doctor working at the hospital.

"I don't believe you," said Noah bluntly "You don't look like a doctor to me!" Of course, wearing a bed sheet would kill my professional image!

I was taken aback, not to say insulted and flustered, and could only answer, "Well I am!"

"What's a first degree heart block?" he shot back.

"Prolonged P-R interval," I answered correctly.

Clever I thought, a question a nurse would not likely know but a medical student would. The music ended and I retreated to join Melodie, who was talking with my new colleague Rob. I never did speak with Noah again as he soon returned south for further studies. Some years later I heard that he had become a respected surgeon.

"I'll just stand here with you," I said to Rob, "to ward off unwanted attention from the many keen young men who don't really interest me."

"Sure," answered Rob. He was going to be a good friend; he already had his eye on a pretty nurse just finishing her evening shift, who would soon join him at the party.

The evening progressed, the noise increased, the wine flowed and grapes were flying as jolly party goers started throwing them around. The young men and women were getting very friendly and the floor was getting very sticky from smashed fruit!

"It's starting to look like a real Roman orgy," I said to Melodie.

"I don't think I want to stay to witness the next part of this story," she answered.

I agreed and we slowly made our way to the door and stepped out into bright daylight, the orange sun hovering above the northern horizon. It was around one in the morning. We walked along the wooden sidewalk to our apartments, wearing our bed sheet togas. I wondered if Robert Service would have ever imagined such a strange sight when he penned his famous poem of strange things done in the midnight sun...

Mid-Arctic Clinic Tour: Churchill, August 1973

After I had been working in Inuvik for less than two months, the Zone Director called me to his office. He was an older doctor with administrative and public health training, and was my supervisor.

He said, "You were hired as an extra doctor this summer because the doctors of Fort Smith were threatening to resign, but they have been persuaded to stay for the moment."

Fort Smith, I learned, was a larger town some 800 miles to the south east.

"Now that the other doctors in this hospital are back from their holidays," he continued, "We have decided to send you on a tour of the eastern arctic. They have not seen a doctor in many months."

"Yes, sir," I said. I was surprised but had no choice in the matter.

I was to be stationed in Churchill, Manitoba along Hudson Bay and would fly to the different villages along the coast. I would stay a few days at each nursing station, seeing patients pre-screened by the nurse practitioner who lived there all year long. I should be back in a month, he calculated.

I packed my bags and said goodbye to Melodie, who was leaving to return to BC since her year in the arctic was over. She had hoped to meet a young man and get married but such was not the case, so she was taking her search elsewhere. I lost contact with her and never did learn about her fate. I can only hope that her quest was successful.

I left Inuvik the next day, flying to Edmonton, Alberta then to Churchill, Manitoba, another 900 miles away. It was a wonderful opportunity to see more of the Arctic and I looked forward to new adventures. An agent of Health and Welfare met me at the airport and took me to a room in an old army barracks. The structure was built to defend the north during World War II. It would be my home base during the medical tour.

Churchill was a bleak, wind blown place with large grain storage buildings. Grain was brought from the prairies and loaded into large freighters to be shipped overseas. The town was also renowned for its white polar bears, which could usually be seen rummaging through the garbage dump. I drove around looking for polar bears one evening, but they were all hiding and I never did see them. I did not regret their absence as it seemed to me that it would be undignified to see those magnificent animals digging in the garbage.

The Health and Welfare agent arranged my flights and gave me the itinerary to visit seven settlements along the coast. I had to be prepared for low lying fog and drizzly rain that would sometimes delay flights for several days. This weather was very common in late summer and we were now into August. Days were already getting shorter and cooler.

Every town that I visited was very different from the others, but they were all situated beyond the tree line and inhabited by Inuit people. Many vivid moments remain in my mind and I will describe a few.

Tundra Walk: Eskimo Point, August 1973

The first village that I visited was Eskimo Point (now known as Arviat), a fully Inuit village along the west coast of Hudson Bay. The nursing station had two resident nurses who were always very busy. Clinic days were full of patients and very long, but low key. The patients spoke no English at all and taking a medical history was most laborious. We worked through a translator, who tended to be a local school student. I listened to the rhythms and sounds of the Inuit language, trying to develop familiarity so I could learn some words just as I had learned some Cree words in Fort George.

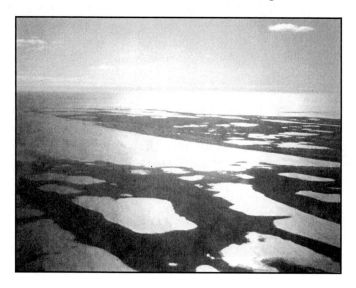

Hudson Bay – the great northern sea.

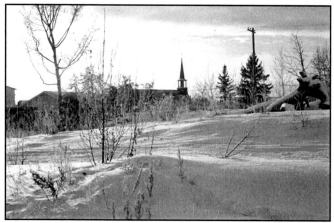

Fort Smith.

"Where does it hurt?" I would ask.

The interpreter would then say what sounded to me like 25 long words. The patients would then answer what sounded to me like 10 long words.

Then the translator would say, "Here," and simply point to the stomach of the patient.

Finally the clinic ended and after our supper, nurse Frances asked if I'd like to join her on an outing along with two of her friends, Debbie and Sean. They were students from University of Manitoba doing summer research, and were heading out onto the tundra to test their instruments.

They were in the village for a few weeks to study the conditions of the flora and fauna of this relatively unknown land. Annie, the other nurse, would stay behind in case some medical assistance was needed by the villagers.

Wearing rubber boots and light jackets we set out walking to the west of town. The land was very flat along the shores of the Hudson Bay and there was not a tree in sight. This truly was the barren tundra. The ground was covered by thick mosses and lichens with small bushes less then one foot tall. Our feet sank in the springing vegetation. We walked and walked for perhaps an hour. The horizon was flat in all directions; the brown reddish land was featureless. The town shrank as we walked and yet remained reassuringly stationary on the horizon.

A light wind blew from the west and I could easily imagine the flat land totally white and endless in winter, with only the inukshuk providing any kind of reference. These sculpture-like piles of large stones were built by the ancient Inuit to mark the land and help them find their way. I could feel the great loneliness of this wild featureless land, which seemed similar to how I imagined the windswept plains of an alien planet like Mars.

Finally we stopped. Debbie and Sean had reached their instruments and were taking some readings.

It seemed to me that there was only a small opportunity for life in this land, and that lay within the two feet between the permafrost over the rocks of the Canadian Shield and the great gray sky. This few inches of soil never fully melted in the short summer. Hardy small plants and wildflowers remained stunted and trees turned into short bushes less than two feet tall.

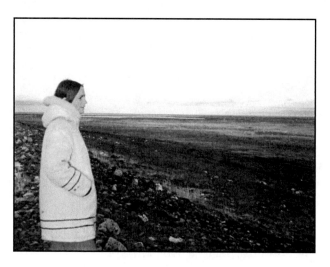

The vast tundra at the edge of town.

We could still see the village far away, small in the distance. I kept checking. I did not want us to get lost in the endless tundra.

Once their measurements were complete, Debbie and Sean picked up their readings and we started back on the long straight walk to the village on the horizon, a radio antenna with a small red light guiding our way. Never did the light from the nursing station look so inviting to me. Dusk was falling on the forbidding land and the short arctic summer was coming to a close. Darkness made daily gains over the pleasant northern daylight hours.

Back at the nursing station, Frances checked what was happening in the clinic and said to me, "Annie has a patient that showed up an hour ago and is having a baby, perhaps you would like to attend?"

"Yes of course," I answered and quickly washed my hands and put on a gown and some gloves.

I entered the dimly lit birthing room where Annie, a trained midwife, was sitting by the bed of a quiet Inuit woman.

"This is her third child," Annie said to me.

"I'll just sit here and assist you," I said, staying behind.

Within another contraction, slowly, without a sound, a beautiful large dark haired Inuit baby was gently brought into the world. This birth felt quiet, intimate, un-medicated, natural and beautiful. It was totally different from the births at the hospital where I had trained, which were noisy, medicated and bathed in harsh lights overseen by bad tempered senior doctors who used many surgical instruments.

This northern birth is really how giving birth should be, I thought to myself, it is the ideal that all women should experience. Yet few women were as fortunate as this Inuit mother in their deliveries.

The next day I returned to Churchill to wait for another trip, but the picture of that beautiful natural birth remains linked in my memory to the mysterious summer tundra of the arctic.

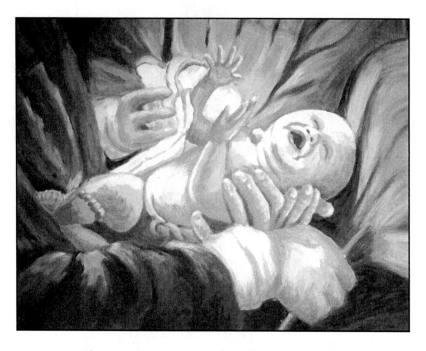

"First Breath" 18"x24" acrylic painted by the author.
Published in the Canadian Medical Association Journal April 18, 2000.

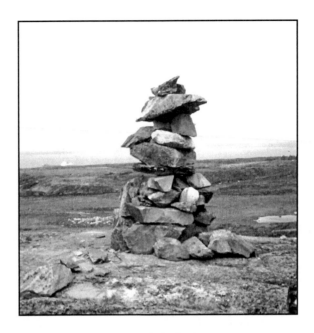

Inukshuk.

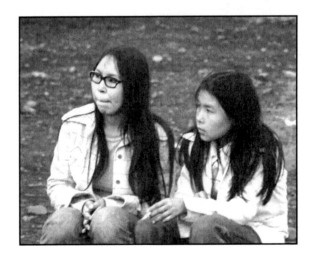

Inuit girls.

Arctic Clinic Afternoon: September 1973

It was a beautiful late summer day with a strong steady wind blowing across the bare tundra. I had just finished two quiet clinic days at Whale Cove, a rocky hamlet where the people spoke no English and long translations were necessary. The days were not easy for a green doctor but I quite enjoyed meeting the legendary Inuit people who lived close to the land.

As soon as I flew to my next destination, the nursing station in Rankin Inlet, the nurse said, "Dr. Lacroix, we have a call from the nurse at Chesterfield Inlet. They want you to come over right away. They have a small child with a plastic wheel from a toy stuck up his nose! They have tried everything and it won't come out. They want you to come over and remove it!"

I hesitated for a second and then said "I guess so." I did not relish the thought of trying to remove a foreign body from the nose of a small screaming child. But as the only doctor for hundreds of miles in all directions I was obligated to do my best.

I walked to the river where a chartered plane waited. It was a sparkling blue Turbo Beaver on floats, the classic bush plane of the arctic. At least this part was going to be pleasant and interesting I thought.

I climbed aboard with the pilot. The plane slowly taxied away from the dock, turned into the wind and, with a roaring display of power and a great splash of water, easily took off. We flew along Hudson Bay, close to shore.

There were no trees, only the small bushes and large rocks of the famous Canadian Shield. The desolate brown landscape extended as far as the eye could see from a couple of thousand feet in the air.

The next village was less than thirty minutes away so we were soon landing in the river and coasting to the dock.

The nurse met us there and said, "Doctor, thank you so much for coming over but the emergency has been cured! About ten minutes ago, the little child sneezed and the plastic wheel flew out of his nose! You can go back now!"

I must admit that I felt relieved. The wind had picked up and there were white caps on the deep blue water. The sky was still totally clear. The pilot turned his plane around and the two of us flew back to Rankin Inlet in his beautiful plane. It was a most pleasant and memorable way to pass a clinic afternoon.

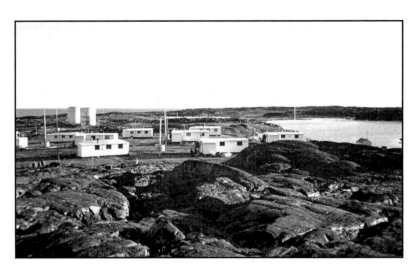

Whale Cove, 1973.

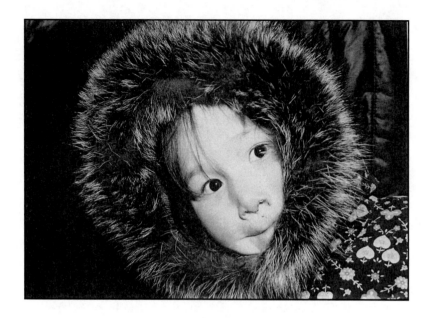

Wasted Arctic Youth: Rankin Inlet, 1973

The leaves covering the ground started to turn red and gold as the end of summer approached; beautiful sunny days were becoming scarce and more precious. Rankin Inlet was a large village where I spent several days, including many hours of translation, in order to see all the people that needed medical attention.

The nursing station, situated on a low hill, overlooked the whole town and the blue waters of Hudson Bay. One evening after we had finished our clinic and our evening meal, I looked through the picture window at the activities in the town below. The area was very rocky with no trees in sight; we were beyond the tree line. Several telephone or electricity poles stood in piles of large rocks surrounded by heavy four feet high corrugated steel circular enclosures. Since the land was rocky and permanently frozen, structures could not be dug into the ground.

I noticed there were very few cars in the town. A nurse called Dorothy was standing with me watching several young people riding back and forth on small motorcycles. We followed their movements as the sun went down low in the northwestern sky.

Suddenly one of the motorcycles headed straight for a telephone pole. We watched in slow-motion horror as the motorcycle hit the corrugated iron barrier and the young man's head, wearing no helmet, crashed into the hard steel.

"Oh my God!" cried Dorothy.

We both ran the half-block to the injured man lying on the ground. We were the first to arrive. As I bent over, I noticed that he was unconscious, not moving at all. I touched his forehead. There was no blood but I could feel a depression on his skull the size of an orange. He had a depressed skull fracture, which is a very severe head injury, and I knew right away that he did not stand a chance of survival. We were 500 miles from the nearest hospital and perhaps 1000 miles from a neurosurgeon.

"Get a stretcher!" Dorothy yelled to the nursing station handyman who had just arrived on the scene.

I smelled alcohol on the young man's breath, and instantly knew the cause of his erratic behavior. Within the few minutes, the wounded young man was carried to the nursing station. As I hurried along beside him, helping with the stretcher, he took his last breath before we even reached the door. We placed him in a bedroom in the nursing station where his family could come to see him.

He was a young Inuit man only 23-years-old. His family was devastated and much loud crying ensued, as was the local custom in grieving. The local RCMP arrived to investigate and the local priest to help them deal with this tragedy.

The next day the young man's second family arrived from the fishing camp with the same deep grief. In many Inuit villages, babies were adopted back and forth between families in what was called an open adoption. If the family had only daughters, they might adopt the son from another family who had many boys. There were probably other subtle reasons that we Klabluna (white people) did not really understand. This young man had been adopted following this ancient custom. Both families considered him their son and both were terribly upset.

The next day I said, "Dorothy, how can this young man smell of alcohol when the only store in town is the Hudson Bay store?"

I had seen this small store and knew that it only sold staple food, a few canned goods and no fresh fruits or vegetables.

"The government brings in alcohol on subsidized flights," Dorothy answered sadly.

I was horrified. "How can this be?" I exclaimed, "Alcohol will destroy these people!"

I was outraged. This was not right! I knew I must do something.

A few days later, I flew back to Churchill and my room in the barracks. I could not get this young man out of my mind. I sent a long handwritten letter to my superior, Dr. Coleville, in Edmonton, deploring the ravages of alcohol on the people of the arctic. My letter went unanswered but I have never forgotten this young man nor his death in the midnight sun.

Double Pneumonia:
Chesterfield Inlet, September 1973

After a few days in Churchill, my next flight was to Chesterfield Inlet, a small village located still further north along Hudson Bay. We arrived safely, but the weather had turned and a large low pressure system was moving over the area. Heavy grey clouds rolled over the bleak rocky lands, pushed by great strong winds.

The rain tapped loudly on the window of the quiet room in the Chesterfield Inlet nursing station. The only sound was the harsh cough coming from Nelly, the only patient. The nurse practitioner, Teresa, poked her head in and said to me, "I want you to see this patient. She is a 34 year old Inuit woman, four months pregnant, and has a terrible cough. She has six children at home already."

I walked to the clinic's patient bedroom and looked at a pale and tired woman who looked much older than her stated age. I had observed that the native women were very beautiful as teenagers but seemed to age very quickly as multiple pregnancies and weight gain took its toll.

I examined Nelly. She was feverish and, pressing my stethoscope gently to her chest, I could hear rales and creps as we called them. It was easy to diagnose "double pneumonia" as the old doctors used to say.

"She's very sick and we have to get her to a hospital," I said to Teresa.

My rotating internship following medical school was serving me well; I could readily diagnose and manage most illnesses I was encountering at this point, and as I was the only doctor available, I was determined do my best to help these people.

"We'll have to call a med-evac," replied Teresa.

Teresa phoned for a plane and returned, saying, "They can't come today but will try tomorrow." It was the news I had expected; a glance outside showed heavy fog moving inland from the large cold Hudson Bay.

An hour later Teresa came to the clinic's exam room, where I was seeing some children, and said, "Bad news, Nelly has started to get labour pains."

I finished the clinic and then sat with Nelly for a while. Sure enough the contractions were coming two minutes apart. We knew that the baby did not stand a chance of survival; at four months of pregnancy, it would be a miscarriage.

Nelly said nothing. She was stoic, as most native women are, but could not suppress the harsh coughing from her body. Nelly's face changed a bit between bouts of coughing and Teresa and I could tell that she felt like pushing.

We washed our hands and dressed in green gown and sterile gloves. I checked her cervix and found it dilated, with a bulging bag of waters. She would pass the fetus soon.

Finally the amniotic sac came out of Nelly whole. It was a transparent balloon about six inches in diameter. Teresa and I stared in wonder at the beautiful miniature baby moving around and floating in a liquid world that would surely burst at any moment. The ball rested in a small bowl and we did not want to disturb it.

"Your baby is too small to survive, Nelly," I said as I showed her the bowl.

Then a thought crossed my mind. Most native people were Roman Catholic in this town, as were Teresa and I.

"Do you want the baby baptized?" I asked Nelly.

"Yes," she replied simply.

Gently, Teresa and I took the bowl to the sink and waited a few seconds. Just as it burst, I sprinkled a few drops of water on the tiny head and murmured, "I baptize you in the name of the Father, the Son and the Holy Ghost."

Teresa joined in, "Amen."

The baby's movements stopped without even taking one breath from lungs that knew only liquid and were not mature enough to breathe air.

The next day the weather improved a bit and a DC-3 plane arrived to take Nelly and me to the hospital in Churchill. Two local men, relatives of Nelly, carried her to the nursing station truck. Teresa drove to the landing strip, where the DC-3 was waiting. After we tucked Nelly onboard with the help of the pilot, we said a hasty goodbye.

With much noisy shaking and rumbling we took off under dark threatening skies. It was a two hour flight and very bumpy, with poor visibility over the bleak land.

The plane carried barrels of fuel located just beside us as part of the cargo. They were tied securely as we were tossed back and forth but we could still smell the strong distinctive odor. I normally have a strong stomach in planes but this time, with the gas fumes and the constant movement, I was feeling nauseated myself. Nelly kept coughing and I was concerned that she might hemorrhage and not survive the trip. Indeed I was concerned about everyone's survival since rushing med-evac planes have been known to crash in the wilderness. The co-pilot came to tell me that the Churchill landing strip was fogged in and we might have to continue to an alternate airport at Norway House, another bumpy two hours further south.

I must admit that I wondered if this was my last flight, if my luck had run out and if my nine lives were all gone. There was nothing to do but silently pray.

Daylight was fast fading and rain was pelting the plane. In breaks between the foggy clouds, I could see tall evergreens on the ground. We must be close I thought.

After much more shaking, we started to descend and finally touched down between the clouds on a runway that looked to me a lot like Churchill. We had not landed in Norway House after all. Joy and relief filled my heart!

There had been a break between the rain clouds and we had managed to arrive at just the right time. It felt almost like a miracle. On seeing the tired looking faces of the two pilots who had worked so hard, I knew that they felt relieved and grateful too.

I escorted Nelly to the hospital, then returned, exhausted, to my room in the barracks, safe and sound. As I drifted into deep sleep to the sound of the pouring rain, I felt certain that I was lucky to be alive. So was Nelly. She recuperated well and within a couple of weeks, made a much smoother flight back to Chesterfield Inlet and her grateful family.

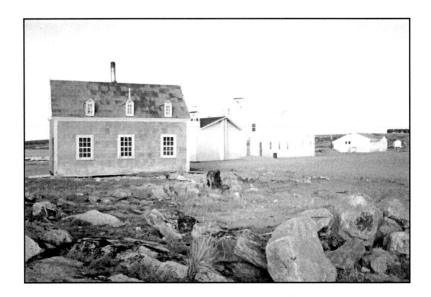

Chesterfield Inlet.

Great Blue Inland Sea: September 1973

It rained steady for five days in late September. Dark clouds hugging the trees prevented any planes from flying along the Hudson Bay coast. The few deciduous trees around Churchill had turned gold and winter would not be far behind. I had just returned from an uneventful four day trip to Baker Lake and was waiting for the weather to clear. Like the chill in the air, I felt a sense of urgency to finish my arctic tour before the freezing weather arrived.

There were still two remote arctic villages left to visit and only then would I be scheduled to return to Inuvik. My only contact with my employer Health and Welfare was the agent stationed in Churchill who arranged my trips. I waited in the plain barrack houses near the airport where I stayed between these flights. Those days were lonely for me. I knew no one and would not be there long enough to get to know any other travelers.

Finally the clouds parted and a cool sunny day arrived. I left for the airport where a sleek twin engine Lamb Air Cessna 401 had been chartered for me. Mr. Lamb was a quiet middle-aged man and a good pilot. We took off and quickly gained altitude, leveling off at 8,000 feet over the sparkling deep blue water of the great Hudson Bay. I sat beside the pilot. We had no other passengers.

The expanse of water reached beyond what my eyes could see and we soon lost all sight of land. I could not help but think that my life hung in the balance of these two piston engines, machines that could break at any time as machines are known to do. We would disappear forever under the great sea with barely a ripple on its cold surface.

The same fate had befallen the famous Henry Hudson only a couple of hundred years before. In his small boat, he did not have a chance.

Yet the beauty of the vast scenery, the steady loud noise of the engines, the sun in the rare deep azure sky and the calm expression on the face of Mr. Lamb all served to reassure me. I had a good feeling about this trip and just relaxed and enjoyed the view.

After a couple of hours we reached Coral Harbour, an Inuit village, the name of which made me wonder how coral might be located in such a desolate place. I had no time to ask, as a busy clinic waited for me at the two-nurse nursing station. I saw many patients for the rest of the day.

The pilot stayed overnight to fly me to Repulse Bay the next day, an even smaller and bleaker windblown hamlet. The low mosses and lichens wore their fall colours of red and gold, noticeable between the gray rocks.

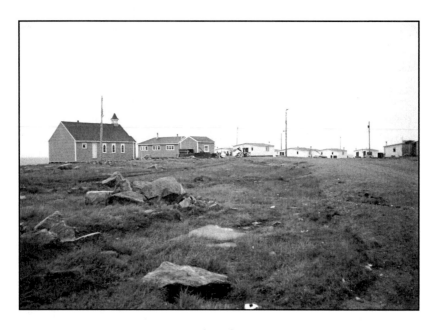

Coral Harbour.

The lone nurse paraded many patients in front of me in rapid succession for they had not seen a doctor in many months. There were a dozen children with congenital heart disease - malformed hearts from birth. A few families suffered from a rare condition called megalo corneas, where the corneas of the eyes are enlarged and lead to vision problems.

The adoption custom was widespread among these isolated people and they had little regard for consanguinity (blood ties). They seemed to me to have lost track of how everybody was related. Bad recessive genes were concentrated by close relative marriages in a small population. It was a very interesting population, I reflected. Humanity needs diversity in their gene pools. The ancient Inuit traveled over many hundreds of miles in search for food, a fact which no doubt contributed to maintaining healthy genes. I quite admired their strength, endurance and their amazing skills of survival.

By the end of the afternoon the weather was holding. Mr. Lamb and I once again climbed 8,000 feet into the sky over the great inland sea of Hudson Bay and safely returned to Churchill.

My journey in the middle arctic was now complete. It had been a most memorable and fascinating time but I missed my colleagues and new friends. The next day, I flew back to Inuvik, winter weather following closely behind.

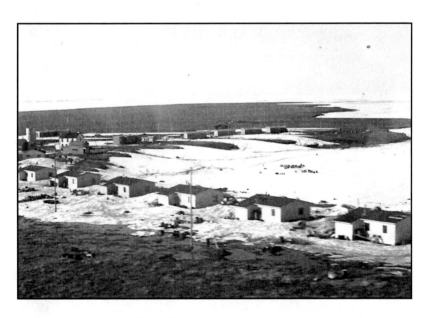

Coral Harbour from the plane.

THREE

Outpatient Clinic: October 1973

When I returned to Inuvik after my six week tour of the eastern Arctic, the eccentric French surgeon was gone and had been replaced by Roy Laine, a very nice soft spoken man in his thirties who had brought his wife and small child with him from Kingston, Ontario, where he had graduated from Queen's University.

We assisted him on many surgical cases. Roy was hard working, careful and competent. He was trained in general surgery only, not the specialties and quickly evacuated cases that he felt were beyond his level of training. General surgery means abdominal surgery such as appendectomies, gallbladder removals and bowel surgeries. It also includes removal of moles and lumps, wound repair, breast cancer surgery and perhaps Cesarean sections. The specialties are gynecology, orthopedics, heart surgery, brain surgery and eyes, ears, nose and throat surgery, to name a few. Roy was well respected by all the doctors and nurses.

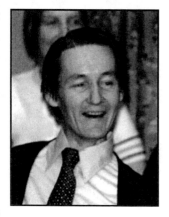

Surgeon Roy Laine.

Winter soon engulfed the land and as much as we had enjoyed the total summer sunlight, we now had to endure total winter darkness.

Indeed winter is the main season in the arctic, occupying a full nine months of the year. The early and middle parts of the winter were dark and so extremely cold that our main recreation was walking or taking a taxi downtown to the grocery store or to the two local restaurants.

We also sometimes gathered at a local pub called The Mad Trapper to meet friends and share local cheer. Late winter was our favorite time for outdoor activities as daylight hours increased and temperatures rose to only 10 or 20 degrees below zero. This was snow shoeing and cross country skiing time. Local people participated in the winter games, and the hospital hosted a fun curling tournament.

On one particularly busy day during my first winter in Inuvik, after visiting half a dozen patients in the hospital, I walked over to the outpatient department near the emergency department. We were holding our monthly Pap test clinic where local women would come to get a pelvic examination and screening for cancer of the cervix. The clinic was heavily booked; word had got out that there was a female doctor in town.

After the clinic ended, I had a hot lunch at the cafeteria and then walked to the office. I was called back to emergency a couple of times to see newly arrived patients. We called them walk-ins in those days.

Back in the physicians' office, the phone rang. We had no personal phones or pagers in the mid 1970's. Pagers had not reached our arctic hospital, though they were available in the south.

"Hello, Dr. Lacroix here," I answered.

"Dr. Lacroix, this is Chipo," the voice said.

Chipo was a competent British-trained midwife from Zambia who had just arrived in Inuvik. She was short, slim and cheerful, and her skin was a beautiful chocolate brown; a source of wonder to the local native people.

Chipo said in a calm voice, "Please come right away, we have two women in labour and they are almost 'fully.'"

Fully meant that the cervix was almost fully dilated and delivery was imminent.

"I'll be right there," I answered as I dropped the receiver into its cradle and ran down the hall for the case room, which for some reason always seems to be built at the far end of any hospital where I have worked.

The case room was just off the maternity ward and Chipo said, "There are no other doctors available, you are the only one."

Chipo was still very calm. I knew that Roy was operating. Rob, the other new doctor was assisting, and Bill was putting the person to sleep. Bill had taken extra training in anesthetics and prided himself on his careful patient work.

They were in the middle of the case. Stuart, another young doctor originally from Australia, was away visiting the patients of his village, Fort McPherson. I was the only doctor to cover obstetrics and emergency cases in our small hospital.

Chipo said, "I'll take this patient," pointing to one patient's bedroom, "and you can take that one."

"Sure," I said, putting on the green gown mask and gloves.

Just as the baby's head was starting to come out the lights in the birthing room went out.

"The generator is acting up again," said Mary, the nurse assisting me, "I'll get a flashlight."

The delivery room was fairly well lit from the window, but another light would be welcome while sewing up any vaginal tears and checking the baby. The births were totally normal and within an hour, two healthy infants had joined this world.

I hoped that the surgery had not been disturbed and was glad to learn that they finished the case just prior to losing the light.

I finished my patient file charting and noticed that it was almost six in the evening. It was already dark and as I walked home to my small apartment to rest and prepare for another day, I felt tired but exhilarated from the excitement of my work.

Northern Tragedy: November 1973

The winter was very dark and cold in November 1973 with the thermometer often hitting forty or fifty below zero. It was my first weekend on call at Inuvik General Hospital and now that I had returned from the eastern arctic, I felt that I was finally really part of the medical staff. I covered calls at our fifty bed hospital, admitted patients and cared for any other patient that came through emergency.

It was a daunting task for a greenhorn doctor. If needed, I could always phone one of the other three or four doctors in town who were off for the weekend. However, I was keen to prove that I was as good as any of them and could handle the situation. I had just finished visiting the half dozen children in the pediatric ward when the nurse said, "There is a call for you from the RCMP."

I took the phone and answered, "Dr. Lacroix speaking."

Lianne Lacroix

"This is constable Mike Peterson," said a deep voice, "There's been a house fire in Fort Good Hope and two people were killed."

I was speechless.

"We are bringing the bodies over to the hospital and we would like you to have a look at them."

Stunned, I said, "Yes, okay."

It was my duty as doctor on call. I did not look forward to the afternoon.

Constable Peterson arrived with the lay (non-medical) coroner, a local person from the village. An orderly took us down to the morgue at the end of one hospital wing. I had never been there before, but felt that I could handle the situation since we had spent a whole year dissecting a body in our first year of medical school.

The constable gave me the names of the victims. They were a young couple in their middle 20s. Perhaps their wooden stove had caused the fire. Perhaps they had been drinking and were careless. When the neighbors noticed the fire, their small wooden house had been engulfed by flames and nothing could be done to help them. Their two young children were spending the night at their grandmother's home and were spared this fate.

The orderly opened the large fridge doors and we looked at the charred remains. They looked like two featureless manikins whose bodies were completely burnt black. I stared in horror. I had assisted at an autopsy or two and spent a year dissecting the cadaver, but these were not people whom I knew anything about.

But this burnt young woman had been my patient. I had seen her only two weeks before for contraception advice. She was attractive and full of life. Now, she was dead, gone, reduced to charred remains.

I was engulfed by the horror of it all. I wanted to scream and run away, but I was a doctor trained to shut down my emotions so that I would retain my scientific logic and clear mind. This was not fair. This woman would never be able see her children grow up. The finality of it all was overwhelming. I am sure the other people with me felt the same way.

We stared in silence for a few minutes or perhaps just a few seconds while all these thoughts and emotions ran through our minds.

Then behind me, I heard a dull thud. I turned around to discover that the male coroner had fainted and fallen on the floor.

This provided a diversion. They orderly ran to get a stretcher and we took our living patient to the emergency department, where he quickly recovered.

The next day, I continued to visit patients on the ward of the hospital.

Constable Peterson phoned again.

"Dr. Lacroix," he said, "We would like to have a sample of blood from the deceased to check their blood alcohol."

I was horrified. "I don't think I could do that," I answered, "Their blood vessels are all burnt off, they're all gone."

"We usually get the blood from the heart in cases like this," he answered.

I could not refuse. "Okay," I said, and then I sat down. I was not sure I could do it.

I told myself that I was a doctor and had no choice but to steel myself and proceed with the onerous task. I would wait until constable Peterson showed up in the afternoon so that he could take the sample with him to the police lab, that is, if I managed to get a sample. I went to the cafeteria, but could not eat very much. Then I walked back to the office and found Bill, the chief of staff, catching up on paperwork with his dog, Gus, under his desk.

I told him about this unusual request from the RCMP and my reluctant, but determined will to comply.

"I'll go," he said matter of factly.

Relief and gratitude flooded my heart. "I would be so grateful," I exclaimed, "Thank you so much."

I was to learn later that Bill had taken two years of pathology after his internship. For him it was a Sherlock Holmes mystery to be studied scientifically that the truth would be uncovered. I was relieved to not look at those blackened human remains again.

As I walked back to my small apartment that night, I thought how wonderful it was to work with a team of dedicated and helpful colleagues. We were saving some lives and doing our best to help people. We helped with births and we helped with deaths. We did what we could. We did not think of ourselves as heroic but as upholding the ideals of our profession, on the edge of civilization in the high arctic.

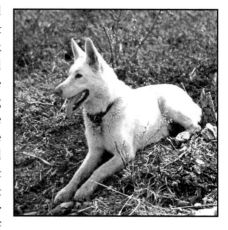

Gus, Bill's dog.

Tiny Christmas Tree: Fort Smith, December 1973

It was early December, and winter was quickly reclaiming the arctic lands. Every day the sun traveled across the sky at a lower angle until it soon remained totally below the horizon. At noon we would see a narrow pink sunrise over the southern sky, but it would quickly turn into a sunset without the sun making an appearance. It was dark for almost 24 hrs a day.

My supervisor from Health and Welfare called me to his office and said, "We have decided to send you to Fort Smith for a few weeks. All the doctors have resigned in that town and they have no doctor at all!"

Then he reminded me again that I had been hired as an extra doctor in July that year because the three doctors of Fort Smith had some dispute with their employer and were threatening to resign. This was the reason I was now being sent to that town.

I was not keen to leave my cozy little apartment and my new friends in the Inuvik Hospital but as an employee I had little choice. I packed my bags, grabbed my snowshoes and stethoscope and caught a plane 700 miles southeast to the town called Fort Smith.

Fort Smith was located well below the tree line and was surrounded by large beautiful evergreens covered in deep snow. The town had been settled a long time ago and had many permanent buildings.

The small hospital was run by a few nursing nuns. Health and Welfare officials lent me a green government car to drive and a plain furnished apartment for accommodation. Every day I drove to a medical office at the edge of town that had been quickly setup inside a small house.

63

I knew no details of the disagreement experienced by the former doctors and had nobody to ask. I was not sure I wanted to know.

It was a most lonely time, associating only with my receptionist who was busy with a family of her own. Christmas morning came and I sat alone in my small bleak apartment with no radio, no TV, no books, no Christmas tree decorations, no gifts, no Christmas food, no friends and most of all, no family. I especially missed my large noisy, cheerful French Canadian family 2000 miles away. I was constantly on call for the town but when I wasn't working, there was nothing to do.

I went to church on Christmas Day and ate Christmas lunch at the small hospital cafeteria. Then I slowly drove the unfamiliar green car back to my apartment. Since Fort Smith was located so much further south than Inuvik, I was looking forward to six hours of daylight, however, heavy clouds hung low over the white snowy town and there was no sun to be seen.

On Christmas afternoon, with nothing else to do, I took my snowshoes and decided to go for a little walk. There was a small wooded area close by on the edge of town and I slowly plodded through the deep snow between the tall pines, feeling down. I carried my camera hoping to take a picture of some kind. I walked further and suddenly the clouds parted and a ray of sun descended, landing on a small perfectly shaped evergreen tree. It was very beautiful; thousands of diamonds sparkled on branches covered with glistening snow.

There it was, I thought, this is my Christmas tree! My spirits lifted immediately and some joy filled my heart. I stood there amazed with wonder and took a photograph. Then the clouds closed again and the sky resumed its bland gray cover. But my spirit had been lifted.

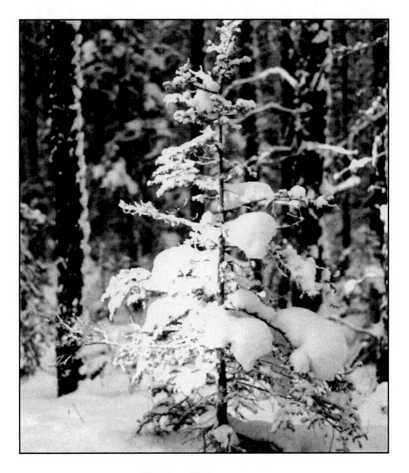

The tiny Christmas tree.

A week later it was New Year's Eve. The phone rang in my apartment. "Dr. Lacroix, this is Sister Anita," the voice said, "please come to the hospital right away, we have a young man who has been shot."

I jumped into my car and drove to the hospital, not too fast, not wishing to get stuck in the deep snow.

The patient was a young native man of Dene Indian ancestry. Sister Anita explained, "It's a Dene custom to shoot into the air to celebrate New Year's Eve and this young man was accidentally shot by a .22 rifle."

I checked the patient. He was lying in bed quietly. He did not seem in pain. He had good vital signs. His blood pressure was stable. He was not in shock. There was a small entry wound in the middle of his abdomen but we could not find an exit wound. We set up an IV.

Even though it was past one o'clock in the morning, I phoned the emergency department in Edmonton to discuss the case with somebody. There was no question of evacuating him in the middle of the night.

"Dr. Carson, surgical resident," said a voice far away.

I explained our situation.

"Is there is anything else we can do?" I asked Dr. Carson.

"You could try probing the wound to see where it goes," he said.

"Thank you for your advice," I said and hung up.

"The doctor in Edmonton suggested that we probe the wound," I told Sister Anita. "We will not do that! I am a family doctor not a surgeon and I don't want to trigger bleeding in the wound and make things worse."

We gave the patient an antibiotic and a painkiller and waited for the morning. The next day we arranged for a medical evacuation to Edmonton. After being treated with surgery, the young man recovered well.

When my six weeks in Fort Smith were nearly over, Stuart Hodgson, the Commissioner of the Northwest Territories (similar to a provincial lieutenant governor), invited me to his house for tea. He was a tall gregarious older man with a good sense of humor. His wife served tea and cookies. I felt an immediate liking for him. There was something about his sense of humor, of not taking bureaucracy or himself too seriously, that was most endearing.

"I want to give you something," he said "to thank you for helping us in Fort Smith when all our doctors had left."

He returned with a beautiful Eskimo carving of a polar bear made from white stone, likely dolomite or marble.

"Thank you so much," I said as I left at the end of the evening, carrying my unexpected Christmas gift.

The white polar bear still watches over me from a shelf in my living room as a reminder of my adventures so long ago.

Nursing Station Visit: January, 1974

I visited the town of Aklavik every month. It was the closest town to Inuvik, a 20 minutes flight and only 40 miles away. Aklavik had been settled before Inuvik, on low-lying land in the Mackenzie River delta, which meant that it was surrounded by the numerous winding channels of the mighty river. Inuvik was settled later on solid land when it was feared that the town of Aklavik would sink into the river in the early 1950's. This fate did not happen and approximately 800 people stayed behind, trapping and hunting in Aklavik.

The Aklavik nursing station was built just across from the runway, no doubt to make medical evacuations easier. It was a large pink two-storey building built above ground on two foot stilts to keep the building above the permafrost. Normally two or three nurses lived there, supported by a local native lady who helped with housekeeping and cooking.

A large clinic room occupied one end of the nursing station. There was an examination table in the middle of the room and large cupboards all around, which contained many medications, especially antibiotics that were given free to the townspeople. Two small patient bedrooms were located at the back, one with a lockable door in case a psychotic patient needed a safe room. The other patient's room was for maternity cases delivered at the nursing station.

The living room of the nursing station always had a half-completed puzzle sitting on a small table and visitors could add a few pieces if they wanted. At 3:00 pm everyday, the staff stopped for tea and a soap opera called "Days of our Lives". The native people really enjoyed that show and the personal dilemmas of the characters in the story. Four staff bedrooms completed the living quarters.

On the lowest floor a large freezer and pantry stored enough food for the whole year since there were no local stores at all. Once a month I would fly to town for two or three days to consult on patients already screened by the nurse practitioners.

One memorable nurse from that town was Liz. She could do anything. She was totally self-reliant and competent, looking after both the patients and the station itself, whether she had to shovel an overflowing septic tank or cook a gourmet meal. Liz could take staple dry foods and frozen ingredients from the giant freezer and make Chinese food! We were all amazed and delighted by her inventions. The rest of the time the local Inuit lady cooked stews and roasts with potatoes, carrots and canned vegetables. Since I had been brought up with a similar diet, I did not notice the lack of fresh foods or salads.

As I visited the Aklavik nursing station every month, the nurses soon noticed my old, well-travelled dark blue parka. The three nurses all wore beautiful golden brown fur parkas with dark or light fur trim, no two exactly the same.

"You should have a new parka made for you, too," Iris, the new nurse said.

The nurses came and went in the nursing stations, many staying for a year or two. However some of them really took to arctic life and never left. Iris was one of those; she eventually married a local Inuit man and found her permanent home in Aklavik.

One day the nurses took me to visit Agnes, an Inuit seamstress, in her home. In one corner of the kitchen was a large table where she would cut and sew the fur garments. The fur was muskrat, a small rodent living in great numbers along the flowing meandering channels of the Mackenzie River delta.

The muskrats were trapped by local men, then the skins were sent to Edmonton for modern tanning and then returned to the local seamstresses for sewing into garments for the local population. At the time there was no negative connotation against using fur for clothes; the Inuit had been doing this for thousands of years.

Agnes took my measurements and had me choose geometric fur decorations on the sleeves and the trim around the hood. The next time I came to town a month later, she presented me with my new fur parka. It cost around $200, which was significant at the time, but it served me very well for all the forty degree below zero days and nights I walked back and forth to the Inuvik Hospital.

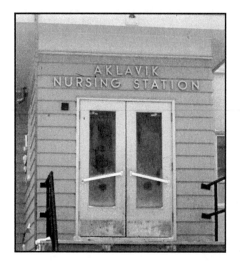

Aklavik Nursing Station.

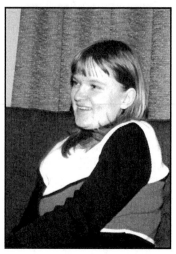

Northern nurse, Liz.

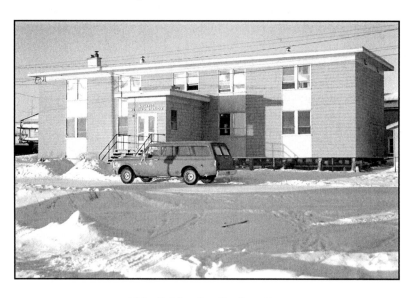

Aklavik Nursing Station, 1975.

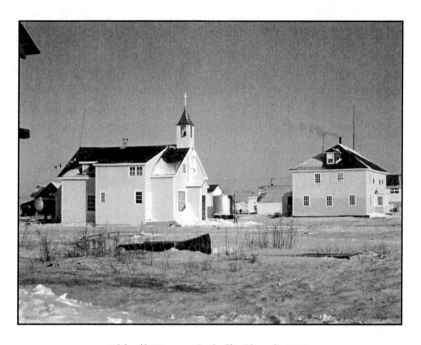

Aklavik Roman Catholic Church, 1975.

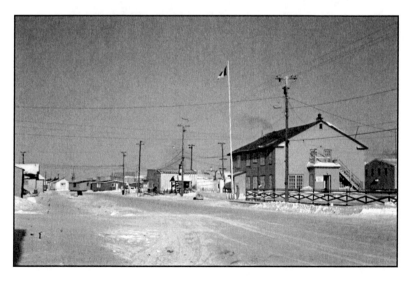

Aklavik street, late winter.

Lianne Lacroix

Aklavik Emergency: February 1974

One winter morning while I was eating breakfast at the Aklavik nursing station, Liz poked her head into the room and said, "Dr. Lacroix, come quickly, we have a man vomiting blood."

I arrived in the clinic room and found a 35-year-old Inuit man looking pale and faint. His alcohol problem was well known. His blood pressure was low, his pulse high, and his stomach tender. We did his hemoglobin on our portable machine and it read 9.0 where the normal is 14-16. The diagnosis was a bleeding peptic ulcer or bleeding esophageal varices. It was a life-threatening situation.

We set up an IV and I told Liz, "We have to call the hospital and get him a med-evac at once."

Just then the phone rang, Liz spoke for a few minutes and returned looking a little pale.

"It's Constance," she said. "She's gone into labor and is coming right over."

I think I looked a little pale myself at that point.

Constance was a nurse who had worked at the clinic the year before. She had married the local school principal and was barely seven and half months pregnant. She was planning to return south for her delivery.

"The baby is only 34-weeks old!" I exclaimed "Very premature."

The other thing that bothered me was that this was her first child and she was a tiny woman, barely five feet tall, and over 30 years old. Shorter women often have difficult deliveries.

Within a few minutes Constance arrived with her husband, Jeff. I examined her. Sure enough, she was 5 cm dilated with bulging membranes and a breech presenting part. The 'presenting part' is a medical term referring to the part of the baby which comes out first, usually the head. In this case, the baby's hips were presenting first, making this birth very complicated.

My heart sank. Here I was, a young GP in an isolated arctic community in the middle of the winter, facing a complicated obstetric emergency with a premature baby and a hemorrhaging man to boot.

A plane could likely get to our village within an hour or two to evacuate the patients. I phoned the hospital and spoke to Bill, the chief of staff, explaining the situation.

Just then Liz yelled back, "Constance's water just broke!"

I knew I could not send her by plane at that point as it would decrease the baby's chance of survival.

"She is better off in the warm nursing station," I told Bill, "At least we have oxygen and IV fluids."

"I'll come right over and help you," said Bill.

Since he was trained in anesthetics, he could do intubation and resuscitation and could help with the baby. It would also be nice to have a colleague for consultation and support. Within 90 minutes Bill showed up by plane and we immediately sent the hemorrhaging man, accompanied by a nurse, on that same plane back to Inuvik for surgical care.

We waited as Constance's labor carried on for another four hours. We sat with her and her husband, who was quite distraught over this turn of events.

Finally Constance's cervix was fully dilated and it was time to push. The baby was small and came out breech and I helped in the traditional manner that I had been taught. As if in slow motion the small bluish body came out with her head last to exit. Bill stood by, ready to receive and resuscitate this small life. He took her to the warm baby bassinet, gave her oxygen and suction.

"It's a girl!" I exclaimed to Jeff and Constance. Tears rolled down their faces. The bleeding was not excessive. We waited for the placenta and waited and waited.

After about an hour I said, "It's not coming, I'll have to remove it manually."

Then I said to Jeff, "You might want to step out," which he did.

"Liz, let's give her IV Demerol and Valium," I said. As soon as the medications coursed through Constance's body, I put on fresh gloves and manually went inside the uterus and removed the placenta. Constance moaned a bit, but she felt no pain and would have no memory of this procedure.

At last all was fine. The small baby called Emily was breathing on her own. We relaxed and all hugged each other with great relief.

By then it was early evening. We called the plane back and returned to the Inuvik Hospital, taking Constance, Jeff, their new baby Emily, Bill and myself. We left the patients under the care of the nurses on the maternity ward at the hospital and we each went to our own homes feeling exhausted and yet exhilarated that all was well.

There was no de-briefing as the process is called now. The next day we carried on as usual and Bill left to visit his two villages, Tuktoyaktuk and Sachs Harbour, as planned. I returned to seeing patients in the outpatient clinic of the Inuvik hospital as always. Yet something had changed.

When I met Bill again a week later, I felt that my respect and affection for him had grown by another degree. When our eyes met in the cafeteria line up, I knew that he felt the same way about me also.

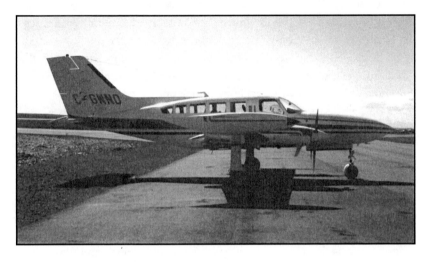

The Cessna 402 often used for med evacs.

Chief of Staff

The chief of staff of a hospital is the senior member of the team who manages the medical affairs of the hospital, making sure that all the other doctors keep the highest standard of care.

Bill had worked at the hospital longer than any of the other doctors and seemed totally adapted to the northern lifestyle, quite enjoying this unusual life.

He did not reveal much about himself but as the months went by I slowly learned more about his story. He came from a small upper middle class Toronto family and was a graduate of the well respected

Toronto University Medical School, where he had also taken two years of pathology studies following his rotating internship.

He was an avid reader of classic literature and collector of antique first edition books. In a quest for adventure with wilderness exploration and camping, he had come to work in the high arctic some four years before. Though he was a city boy, he found the northern lifestyle suited him perfectly. He let his hair and beard grow as many young men did in the seventies and lived with his dog in a bungalow close to the hospital. He had adopted Gus as a puppy and often brought him to the hospital where the faithful and well trained canine waited under the desk while his master visited patients.

I once asked Bill, "I see you always wear a shirt and tie with a white coat in the hospital, why so formal?"

"I know that my long hair can put people off," he answered, "so I wear a tie to look more professional." He was sensitive to his patients and well liked.

Many times I consulted with him on difficult cases and as the months went by he would sometimes even ask my opinion sometimes about some women's health issues.

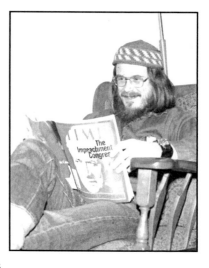

I had a feeling that he had not worked with women doctors before as the medical classes in those years accepted perhaps eight or ten women for sixty or eighty men. I was keen to gain his respect and prove myself competent as a doctor. Sometimes I would go to his

Chief of Staff Bill Sara

house, along with his best friend, the young curly haired dentist, Al. Together we would watch an episode of Sherlock Holmes on the TV or sometimes we went canoeing in the summer or snowshoeing in the winter.

I felt that Bill and I were parallel personalities with many things in common in our work and life, yet our hearts did not meet. As greatly as I enjoyed our friendship, I felt sure that he was not my life partner.

Coppermine Drum Concert: March 1974

As spring arrived, evening light lasted a little longer each day and the sun sparkled like a million diamonds over the deep snow. It was early spring, my favorite time of the year in the arctic. A circumpolar medical conference was being held in Coppermine, an Inuit village along the Arctic Ocean 500 miles east of Inuvik. I was fortunate enough to be chosen to attend this meeting along with Bill.

We left by a Twin Otter plane on skis and after stopping at several villages, arrived at our destination. Coppermine was still buried in very deep snow that almost totally covered the two dozen buildings. Frozen whole caribou meat was hanging outside houses, kept in a natural deep freeze. Dog teams and skidoos were the only mode of transportation.

The last day of our two day conference, all fifteen members of our group were invited to an evening of entertainment by some local villagers. Wearing our heavy parkas, wind pants, seal skin boots and fur mitts, we sat on plain wooden benches in what can only be called a shed – a large un-insulated, unheated plain rectangular wooden building. It was probably the town hall. Half a dozen Inuit men entered to the front of the hall carrying circular drums about two feet wide. Thinly stretched caribou skin covered a narrow wooden frame.

Then the drumming started. Boom, boom, beating simple ancient rhythms that went on and on without stopping, growing louder and louder as the world receded and only the drumming occupied our consciousness.

After about 20 minutes, half the people in our group left and went to bed. I wondered if they had not lived in the north very long. The rest of us, perhaps a dozen people, just sat on the wooden benches hypnotized by the boom! boom! boom! of the drums penetrating our bodies right down to our bones. We felt in a trance, not wanting to move, not wanting the drumming to stop, it went on boom boom boom for perhaps an hour or two. Time had no meaning, and there was nothing else in the world but the constant rhythm of that incessant pleasant drum. I was aware that I was privileged to join a tradition extending back thousands of years to the earliest Homo Sapiens, who were known to have taken part in this very ancient ritual. The drumming bonded us together as a people, to the depth of our earliest most primitive nature. Boom boom continued the Inuit hunters beating on their drums, lost in the legends of their ancestors.

Just as suddenly as it had started, the drumming stopped. No words were spoken; we were beyond words. Slowly we got up from our benches and walked outside to a cold winter night illuminated by millions of stars. Great veils of iridescent pale green and shimmering reds danced across the whole sky from one side to the other. The northern lights offered us one last spectacle as the women from our group walked to their cabin and the men to theirs. That night the arctic had touched my soul in a way that I had not expected. As the snow crunched under my feet, just as it had for the first humans who had ever walked this land, I knew that I have been given a most precious gift.

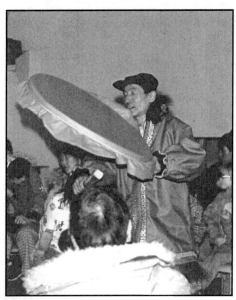

Inuit drummer
and dancer.

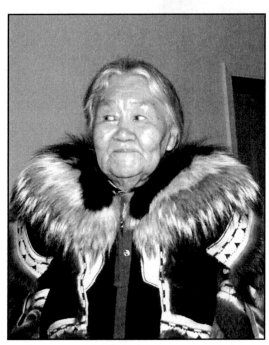

Lianne Lacroix

Winter Incident: Paulatuk, April 1974

One dull winter day, a call came in to the hospital, asking for a doctor to visit the hamlet of Paulatuk, 200 miles northeast of Inuvik along the Arctic Sea. The village was too small to have a nursing station; fewer than one hundred people lived in the desolate area beyond the tree line.

I set off for the community in a chartered Cessna 337. The pilot was named Hans, a man in his late twenties with a northern European accent, who seemed nice enough. We were planning to return the same day, as my friend and colleague Stuart and his fiancée, a nurse, were planning to get married the next morning at the nurses' residence and we had all been invited.

As we were taking off for the two hour flight I noticed immediately that Hans was wearing a light coat instead of the usual heavy arctic parka. I looked in the back of the small six person plane and could not see a parka anywhere. Not good, I thought to myself. While traveling in the arctic, one must always be prepared for emergencies. We could get stuck somewhere or have to land because of a mechanical problem or worse. There was nothing I could do, so I didn't say anything.

I always paid careful attention to planes and flying conditions. During my last two years of medical school, I had taken flying lessons as a hobby and obtained my private pilot license. Although not very comfortable with noisy engines, I quite enjoyed the magnificent scenery from the air.

Soon some twenty small houses huddled together appeared in the great white wilderness. This was the village of Paulatuk. We landed, with no trouble, on the frozen airstrip between the houses.

We were met by an elder of the village and a translator who offered to lead me to see the patients. Immediately Hans wandered off between the houses, attracting the attention of several children who followed behind him. My patient was an elderly Inuit woman who had a fever and a terrible cough. I examined her and after a long back and forth translation of her medical history, there was no doubt she had pneumonia and should return to the hospital with us. The translator asked me to check a few other sick people in the village. I returned the short distance to the runway to tell Hans that I would be another hour before I was done.

I noticed there was a cold wind blowing off the bare frozen tundra. I remembered well my previous trip to Paulatuk when the pilot kept saying "Hurry up, hurry up the plane will freeze" and then start the engines to warm them up every twenty minutes. I had expected Hans to do the same.

I was most surprised to find him playing a game of tag with several children, laughing and screaming all around the plane. This was not very safe. I was very concerned. I advised Hans of our time of departure and returned to the patients. An hour later after checking two more sick children and one adult, I was ready to leave with the elderly Inuit lady.

Hans tried to start the plane and nothing happened. He tried again and again, no luck. "Something must be wrong," he said.

Of course, the engine was so cold that the plane would not start! Anybody who comes from the cold parts of Canada knows that feeling very well.

"I must phone the base," said Hans.

By then, it was getting pretty late in the day and the few daylight hours were long gone. The patient returned to her house and Hans returned, saying, "They cannot come and help us today. We must spend the night."

Again I said nothing. It would not help. But I felt angry and disappointed. There was little chance that I would return in time to attend my friends' wedding. In the arctic, we quickly learn to make the best of things.

Fortunately two different families offered us shelter for the night. I stayed far away from Hans or I might have been tempted to say something unprofessional that I would later regret. The next day around noon a company Twin Otter plane piloted by Murray and carrying a plane mechanic arrived to our rescue.

"I do not know why the plane does not start," said Hans as he walked off with the mechanic.

They took out a special large heater called the Herman Nelson, and reheated the plane, finally managing to get the engine started after a few more hours. The patient and I returned to Inuvik in the Twin Otter with Murray.

When we landed at the base in Inuvik, as my patient was being loaded into the Health and Welfare station wagon, I said to Murray, "May I speak with somebody in charge at the base?"

He introduced me to Mike Zubko, a small very pleasant middle aged man, and the owner of Aklavik Flying Services.

"That pilot is not very safety minded," I said. "I think that you should know what happened. He let the plane freeze up and he was not even wearing a parka," I said.

I normally do not like to complain but I felt that this situation could have been very dangerous and could have ended in disaster. I then detailed the events of the previous day.

"Thank you for telling me," said Mike, "I will take care of it." I then returned to the hospital where the patient settled on the ward with antibiotics and oxygen. By then, it was late afternoon, the wedding was long over and I returned to my apartment grumbling silently to myself.

Several weeks later, I heard that Hans had left town after Mike had encouraged him to resign his flying job. Several months later Hans died in a plane crash in Germany along with several unfortunate passengers.

Black Misery: 1974

It snowed a very fine dry snow all day, making the world vanish in a white frozen cloud. I walked home from the hospital thinking about a patient and asking myself how I could possibly help to make a difference in her life.

Her name was Flossie. She was a 24 year old Dene woman who was the mother of seven children and was now pregnant for the tenth time. She had suffered two miscarriages. I had seen her once for a prenatal visit and she never came back. She had come to the hospital in the evening a couple of times with a sick child; she always looked pale and exhausted and never smiled.

I reviewed the medical files written by the previous doctors who had attended her births. They had given her birth control pills but she forgot to take them. They had suggested an IUD (intra-uterine device) but she came to see us only when pregnant so an IUD could never be inserted. We could understand why she never came to the hospital. She was too busy trying to look after all those children while her husband held a series of menial jobs. They were very poor.

"La misère noire," we would say in French, which translates as black misery.

I had seen such troubles before in families with too many children. Sick mothers could not look after the children and fathers avoided the chaos at home by hiding at the pub.

I was brought up in a devout Roman Catholic family. My religion said contraception was wrong except for the rhythm method, which many couples cannot use successfully. In catechism, which is the teaching of religion to Catholic children, we had been taught to listen to our conscience – the little voice inside our heart that tells us right from wrong. I listened. It said that black misery was wrong. I was sure of that. It said contraception was right, I was sure of that also.

So here was poor Flossie caught in black misery. What could I do to help? I wondered if I could offer to insert an IUD right after her next delivery before she left the hospital. I kept looking through the medical journals for an answer of some kind. One day I found an article written by a doctor in Africa who had the same problem. His maternity patients never came back either. He reported that he was inserting IUD's one week after birth before the women went home. This is what I was looking for, a precedent that I could quote if needed.

Finally Flossie returned to the hospital in good labour. She progressed well and within a few hours gave birth to a beautiful baby girl that she named Minnie.

At the time we kept women in the hospital for five days after a birth.

By the fourth day, Flossie was getting pretty keen to go home.

"If you stay till tomorrow, I can insert an IUD as we discussed. Then you can go home right after," I said, emphasizing the opportunity to 'go home'. I was trying to encourage her to agree.

"Okay," she agreed reluctantly.

The next morning I grabbed an IUD insertion kit from the outpatient department and a Lippes Loop IUD which was available for free. They were "S" shaped, made of white plastic, rather big and came in four sizes from A to D.

I chose size D for Flossie.

With the help of the night nurse, Myra, we positioned Flossie on the foot of her bed and brought over a large spotlight. I did not use a *sound,* which is a thin metallic ruler used to measure the depth of the uterus in order to pick the right IUD size. I was afraid of perforating her tender uterus and was sure that she had enough room for the two inch plastic device. Deep inside slid the IUD with no trouble at all. Her uterus felt like a dark warm cave. Soon we were finished and Flossie went home with her baby.

I did not see her again for three years. Then one day she came to the hospital bringing Minnie, a lively 3 year old who had a sore ear.

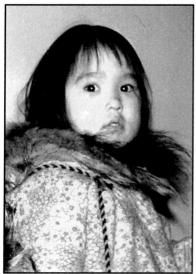

Flossie was not pale, not pregnant, and even smiled! I watched her walk away. The IUD was obviously still inside, doing its job. I felt very pleased. It had all been worthwhile. No more black misery for her. It had been banished by a piece of white plastic in the right place at the right time and her life had been improved.

Inuit child.

85

The Walk Reflection: July 1974

Spring finally came to Inuvik. The snow melted quickly and rain made our streets muddy and slippery. I had just returned from a three week holiday to see my family in Ottawa and continued work at the hospital with the new replacement summer doctors. Doctors at the time did not really sign a contract, instead they gave verbal agreement as to whether they would stay another year. I wondered what to do.

One summer evening as the sun circled around the sky in the land of the midnight sun, I went for a walk. I had now been working for over one year at the Inuvik General Hospital. I was a single woman in my early thirties hoping to soon meet my life companion. I had no luck so far. I had met many new people and several of them had become good friends but nothing more.

I was sure that the person who would share my life lived in my future and not in my present or past. I was searching for a sign as I walked up the deserted gravel road leading to a small lake above the town. I settled into quiet reflection from which I was hoping I could calculate my next course of action.

I walked past the part of town where the trees were sparse and dwarfed following a forest fire in the recent past. In winter our cross-country ski trails crossed this area and travelled over low bare hills to the east.

I sat on a large rock and looked at the lake, focusing on the moment and trying to quieten the voices inside my mind that remind me of daily concerns, worries and the constant details of life. I projected my memory back in time, trying to link to other quiet moments in my life where I had stopped and wondered at my destiny.

Ten years earlier I sat quietly on the sandy shore of a large northern river in Fort George looking at the banks of fog moving in rapidly from the ocean, trying to pierce the veils of mystery surrounding our lives. I tried to imagine my future, which was now my current present. I searched for that moment of clarity where one can see their life in a new perspective. My vision that day remained wrapped in fog, impenetrable.

Now I looked at the skinny trees and the calm sky asking these same questions. Did I belong in this place now? Should I stay here? Where was my life going? Was my life companion waiting for me somewhere else?

I listened for answers, for that little voice inside my mind to speak. I believe that we all have such a little voice of intuition but we are usually too busy to listen.

I have always believed in my own destiny, at being able to navigate the waters of uncertainty to find where I really belong at each stage of my life. I focused on the lavender and purple fireweed growing all around the lake reminding me that the short summer would not last much longer. Soon the low hills would turn gold, red and maroon in one last glorious burst of life before the land turned white again. I could feel the passing of time.

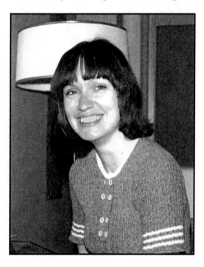

Then a feeling of peace filled my heart and my little voice said not to worry, I would not be alone forever. There was a person out there in the future who would be

Content Inuvik doctor, 1974.

my best friend. He was coming my way in every decision that he made, just as my life was heading in his direction by every decision that I made every day. Have no fear, my little voice said, you are on the right road.

I had always been fascinated by fate—how a series of seemingly trivial events totally change a person's life one way or the other. Many details in our life make no difference at all, yet a few crucial details here and there can change everything forever. Every so often we are faced with a choice, a decision about which road to take, that will make all the difference - although we can only pick these important events and decisions in retrospect.

A calm feeling came over me. I had my answer. The time was getting closer. I could feel it as I walked back to my apartment, confident that I was following the right road of my true destiny, walking one step at a time with the sun shining low in the western sky.

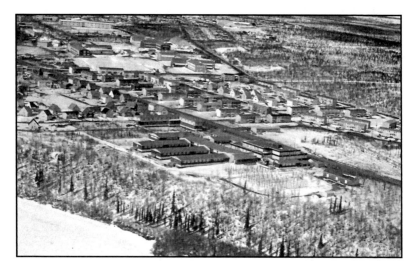

Inuvik, with hospital center front. Photo taken from the air, 1974.

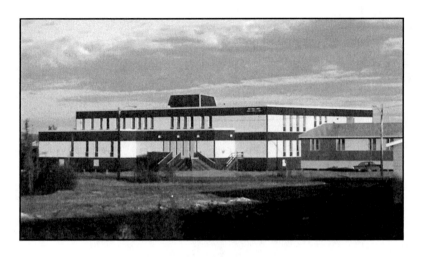

Inuvik General Hospital, 1975.

Roses in an August Snow Storm: August 1974

Our short summer was underway; the hordes of mosquitoes that occupied the wet lands of the Mackenzie River delta fortunately did not bother us too much in town.

I continued to work every day at the hospital, delivering babies at all hours, visiting hospital patients and seeing people at the outpatient department.

One day Corrine, our medical secretary, said, "Dr. Lacroix, I have a message for you. You have a gift waiting for you at the front desk to pick up on your way home."

I walked down the long hall wondering what this could possibly be. At the front desk, the receptionist handed me a large bouquet of perfect, beautiful long stemmed red roses!

Roses in the arctic? I stared in amazement! I had never seen them before in town.

There was a card. Trembling with excitement, wondering which handsome young man would pose such a wildly romantic gesture, I opened the card.

It read, "Dr. Lacroix please accept my apologies, the forms finally arrived and my case is fine, sorry for the bad things I said." It was signed Fred Baker.

I stared for few moments trying to place Fred Baker. Then suddenly, I remembered. He was a patient. He had been working for a gas exploration company and his hand was mildly injured at work. I had filled the Workman Compensation form and mailed them to his company. He had returned to his home in Edmonton.

Two weeks later, he had phoned, asking to speak with me.

He was very angry. "My forms never reached the company," he stated, "You're a no good doctor. Why don't you just go back to your toboggan and dogs!" he yelled and slammed the phone down.

That outburst had bothered me, but I knew the forms were properly filled in. They were likely just delayed in the mail, so I had forgotten about this incident.

So now I carried the precious beautiful roses – from a nutty patient - in my arms, smiling at the incongruity of it all. I opened the hospital door and discovered that it was snowing! It was August yet there was an inch of wet snow all over the ground. Carefully, with my slippery shoes, I walked on the board sidewalk back to my apartment carrying precious bright red roses that seemed to glow in the totally white world. Summer in the arctic with roses and snow!

The roses did not seem to mind the sprinkle of snow and lived gloriously for a week sitting in a jar on my small dining room table. I had no vase. Fred Baker was never heard from again and I never did own any sled dogs.

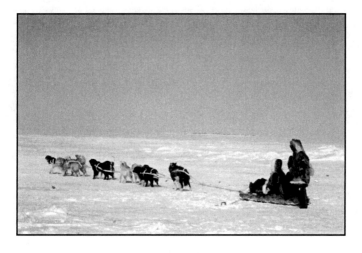

Sled dogs working.

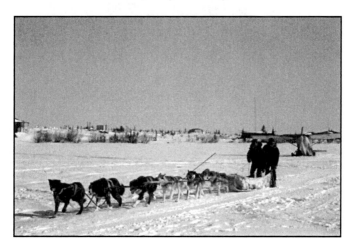

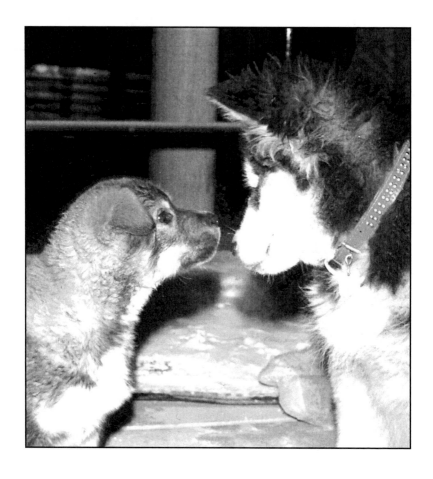

FOUR

New Surgeon: September 1974

The short arctic summer of 1974 ended suddenly as the low hills around the hospital turned gold and copper; splashes of deep red brightened the leaves of the groundcover, and it all seemed to happen overnight. Fire had swept these hills some years before and the sparse evergreens had not yet returned. We felt the cold chill lengthen each morning as winter prepared to return again.

I had returned from a three week visit with my family and felt refreshed and ready to carry on. By the end of the summer Bill left for a six week holiday which would see him hiking with friends in the mountains of Alberta after visiting his family in Toronto. He cheerfully wrote to me that he had met a girl named Shirley and that they were together. By September, he returned to Inuvik, bringing Shirley to work as a nurse at our hospital. She was a lovely, slightly exotic looking woman and I liked her right away. The new couple seemed very happy. Bill's reserve was gone and he was cheerful and smiling all the time.

New doctors arrived as the summer replacement doctors went south. My colleague, Stuart, returned to Australia with his new bride and Rob moved to Edmonton, following the pretty nurse who was now his girlfriend. I verbally agreed to work another year in the arctic and felt that it was the right thing for me to do.

We welcomed to our medical staff Ronald Calderisi, a vibrant young man of Italian descent from Montreal who had graduated from McGill University. He was accompanied by his girlfriend, a delicate looking nurse called Diane. It did not take long for Ronald to adapt to arctic life and to fit very well with the medical staff. He immediately started to visit his villages of Fort Good Hope and Arctic Red River. He was outgoing and cheerful and soon became a good friend.

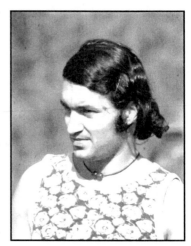

Ron Calderisi.

An 'older' doctor, Maurice, perhaps in his late forties, continued working with us, dispensing folk-wisdom along with his medical advice. I quite enjoyed discussing cases with him and learning many useful medical tips. He was the only doctor that I had ever met who kept count of the babies that he delivered; for each new birth, he would add a tick to a piece of paper taped to his fridge. He wrote in one patient's file that she was his one thousandth delivery as if this was a special badge of honor, which indeed it was.

Maurice came from the southern states, most likely a rural area, I guessed by his drawl. He was cheerful and calm but disclosed very little about himself. He never mentioned having any children, and I noticed his wife, Betty, was much younger. I wondered if she was perhaps a second or third marriage, but never asked.

The other new doctor that fall was named Larry. He was very handsome, but unfriendly, reserved, even cold. He kept very much to himself and befriended only Maurice. I had a feeling that he was hostile to women in general. He seemed to avoid me as much as possible. I was glad to reciprocate.

Our new surgeon, Angelo, arrived during this time to replace Roy who had finished his one year term. We had heard that Angelo was from Italy and had recently worked in Newfoundland.

I first met him one day at the hospital when my colleague, Ronald, said, "Lianne, this is our new surgeon, Dr. Angelo DiStefano."

"Nice to meet you Dr. DiStefano," I replied.

"Call me Angelo," he said.

I shook hands with the fairly nice looking 40-year-old Italian man.

When he heard my name, he said, "Do you speak French?"

"Yes," I answered, "I'm from Ottawa."

He switched to French immediately, and always used that language in our conversations as his Italian-accented French was better than his Italian-accented English.

He seemed the stereotypical Italian to us, intense, passionate, emotional, yet he was a typical surgeon in that he saw the world in black and white. We soon became good friends.

He would meet us every day in the hospital at eight to see surgical patients that we referred to him and perform various scheduled surgeries.

In time he told me that he was separated from his wife, Stella, who lived in Italy with their teenage daughter. They had met at university in Rome when she was doing a degree in chemistry and he was in medical school.

He had done his surgical residency in Detroit, USA while Stella had remained in Rome with their daughter.

My colleagues and I assisted with all of Angelo's operating room cases, and we found him to be an excellent surgeon. He had great compassion for the patients and was very confident in surgical cases whether gynecology, orthopedics, C-sections or bowel surgeries. He seemed especially confident and experienced in the various trauma cases that came to our emergency, such as stabbings and shooting wounds. These were unfortunately all too frequent as alcohol ravaged the local population. He told us that he had been a surgical resident in Detroit during the race riots of the 1960s, which would explain this specific expertise.

The general consensus was that he was by far the best surgeon that Inuvik had ever known, and we were happy to work with him. He helped many people and saved many lives.

Ronald, Bill and I quickly learned to admire Angelo's surgical skill and to enjoy his emotional Italian temperament. Ronald, who especially appreciated Angelo, likely because of their common Italian heritage, said to me a few months later, "I really like assisting at surgery with Angelo. Would you mind if he calls me first, so I would be his permanent assistant when I am in town?"

I answered, "That is fine with me. I would just as soon see the patients in the outpatient clinic."

Surgery was really not my special interest, although I knew it could be intense, dramatic and ultimately satisfying. I preferred obstetrics, gynecology and women's and children's health.

Not everybody, however, liked Angelo. Maurice remained reserved and seemed to question Angelo's credibility. Perhaps Angelo was too exotic for the rural southern-US sensibilities of a person who had not yet been to Europe. As the months went by and the two men shared many patients, Maurice had to admit that Angelo had great diagnostic and surgical skills. I could tell that Angelo was earning Maurice's hard-won respect.

Larry was quietly hostile, which was normal for him. He seemed jealous of all the attention that Angelo attracted around himself, especially the admiring nurses who surrounded Angelo at our local pub, The Madtrapper.

But even though we knew Angelo was now single, he was not attached to any one nurse in particular. He lived by himself in his townhouse and seemed not to care at all what anyone thought about him.

Tourtière: December 1974

The hardest time of the year in the arctic was always the depth of winter, November through February. There was no sun for it was totally invisible below the horizon. At noon, the southern sky would lighten a bit, sometimes turning pink or gold, then darkness would reclaim the land. Temperatures stayed around 40° below zero except when it climbed to perhaps 30° below when snowstorms passed through. The weather was strangely stable, keeping the same cold and darkness for weeks on end. We walked back and forth from our houses to the hospital, which was only a block or two, and we could not cross-country ski or snowshoe since it was unsafe in the dark and cold. Walking the few blocks to the store in town was almost a major expedition.

The only bright spot during the depth of winter was Christmas. To celebrate my first festive season in Inuvik, I decided to make tourtière, a French Canadian meat pie made only at Christmas. All the doctors had been invited to Angelo's house for Christmas dinner, and would each bring a dish; I was happy to share my family tradition. I truly missed my home at Christmastime; my large family would go to midnight mass on the 24th, and on Christmas Day would feast on turkey and tourtière.

It was now the evening before Christmas and I was working on making two tourtière pies. The savory filling of ground pork and veal was simmering on the stove filling my small kitchen with the mild spicy smell of Christmas. For some reason I could not get the pie crust to stick together although I was following the exact recipe that I had made before. I did not know what to do. I tried again and again only to have a crumbled mess remain on my counter.

"If only I could ask someone," I thought, but I was alone.

Just then, the doorbell rang. I opened the door and there stood Santa Claus dressed in a red outfit trimmed with white fur, sporting a long

white beard. Of course it was reasonable to expect Santa since the arctic was so close to the North Pole! I explained my culinary dilemma to him and Santa said, "The air is very dry here and the flour came by boat and could be very dry also. You likely need to increase the water."

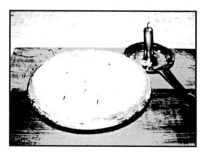

Tourtière: French Canadian specialty.

"Of course," I said, "Thank you, Santa."

I tried again to make the pie crust and this time it held together just fine. I made a note to thank Frank, our hospital pharmacist, for his tip. He had dressed up to make the rounds to invite us all to a children's celebration at the hospital a few days later.

The next day we had a most pleasant meal at Angelo's house and not one hospital emergency disturbed the cheer rarely felt during the deep dark days of winter.

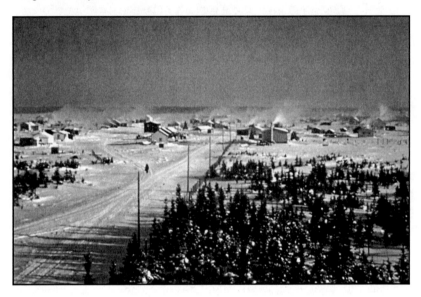

High noon, in the depths of winter in an arctic village.

Roasted Deer: January 1975

The phone rang with that loud mid-1970's jarring ring. Wearing my flannelette nightgown, I jumped out of bed and ran, half asleep, to the hall in front of my bedroom. We did not have portable phones, pagers or cell phones; we had only seen such devices on Star Trek.

"Hello?" I said, trying to chase the cobwebs of sleep from my mind.

"It's Bill," the familiar voice said, "Can you come and assist, we have a case of gunshot wound to the abdomen."

"Sure, be right there," I answered as expected, and hung up the phone. I was not surprised as we were always on call. There were four or five doctors in town but we could all be needed at any time.

It was dark, as usual, and I only realized that it was 4:10 a.m. when I glanced at the clock. I knew it was around 40° below zero outside; a cold that could kill a lightly dressed person in twenty minutes.

I dressed as fast as I could, putting on jeans, a light sweater, wind-pants, a heavy sweater, my muskrat fur parka with fur hood, scarf, fur mitts and big boots. All this for my two-block walk to the hospital.

The cold air woke me up completely. The night was clear and thin columns of smoke rose from the dark houses. My feet crunched on the thin layer of snow covering the wooden sidewalks. It was hard to breathe so I pulled my scarf over my nose to prevent frostbite.

Our one main street was deserted but the low dark hospital buildings glowed with light. I walked through the emergency door and the lone nurse waved a greeting as I started down the hall towards the OR, peeling off the layers of clothing as I went.

Angelo had arrived and was getting ready.

"Hello," he said, speaking to me in French, "This poor man was shot in the stomach, we must open him up." I enjoyed our conversations in French.

Before surgery, Angelo was always calm, confident, and totally focused on the patient. We dressed in green cotton outfits, put paper masks over our faces and scrubbed hands to elbows with special anti-microbial soap. With hands dripping, we walked backwards into the operating room where Anna, the circulating nurse, handed us sterile towels to dry our hands, and then long green gowns and sterile gloves. A circulating nurse is one that is not wearing sterile gowns and gloves, who walks around getting instruments prepared; sort of a gopher for the operating room.

Our efficient surgical nurse, Sadie, was already removing instruments from sterile packets, getting ready to assist. Bill was sitting beside the anesthetic machine putting the patient to sleep. His shoulder length hair was covered by a long green paper cap, which made me think of the neck coverings of French Legionnaires I'd seen in movies.

We all greeted each other with eye contact and a slight nod of the head and started the "case". The patient was a young native man barely 30 years old, who was brought to our emergency by the local RCMP. He was no doubt involved in drinking alcohol when he had been shot by another person, perhaps accidentally or perhaps not. No other details were available. It did not matter to us. We passed no judgment. He was a person in distress, a patient. We were there to help, nothing else mattered.

Angelo opened the abdomen in one smooth motion and explored the intestines looking for damage caused by the bullet, repairing as he went along. I assisted Angelo, holding retractors, and helping as much as I could while Sadie handed us instruments, almost reading our minds as to which one came next.

Angelo inspected the bowel, removing the damaged parts and expertly sewing the ends of bowel back together. His hands were skilled, precise, highly trained. He had performed this procedure many times before. Finally the bullet was removed and the wound was closed. The operation took a long time but the patient would survive.

It was now 7am. Somewhere in the world dawn would be breaking, but not in our part of the world. Today we would only see a reddish streak in the south-facing sky around noon.

It was too late to return to our houses, so we went to the cafeteria for breakfast, doctors and nurses sitting together. We felt exhausted and exhilarated at the same time. We had saved another life. This is why we were here and why we had trained for so many years. We were part of a special team, looking after the health of the 5000 people in our town and the perhaps 4000 people from the regional villages. They were in our hands, and on this day we had honoured that trust.

After breakfast we started another day as usual.

One month later a large parcel covered with brown paper arrived for Angelo in our common office. An elderly native man deposited the parcel on his desk and said, "I want to thank you for saving my son." Then he turned around and left. The parcel contained a large roast from a deer. Angelo invited us all to his house a week later where he cooked the roast, which he had basted with Italian wine. It was delicious.

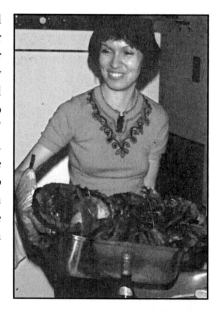

Enjoying roasted venison with colleagues.

Royal Fossil: Colville Lake, April 1975

By April, winter finally showed signs of leaving. The sun shone brightly on deep sparkling snow and hours of sunshine increased daily. I realized that I had now been in the arctic for almost two years.

My colleague, Ronald, was gone on holidays and so I was scheduled to visit his villages of Fort Good Hope and Colville Lake. We had heard that Charles, the Prince of Wales, would visit Colville Lake, and I learned that there was a chance I would get to see him. Although not a big fan of royalty, I was certainly curious.

After I finished seeing the patients at the nursing station in Fort Good Hope, the nurse, Peggy, and I flew to Colville Lake. Peggy was a vivacious grey haired nurse in her early 50s, who quite enjoyed northern life.

Fewer than 100 people lived in Colville Lake and the log cabin nursing station was only occupied when a nurse visited; the hamlet was too small to have a permanent nurse.

The town is located below the tree line, 600 miles southwest of Inuvik. Several buildings were made of local evergreen logs, giving the small village a picturesque appearance on the shores of the great Colville Lake.

The largest building was built like three log cabins joined together. It operated as a fishing lodge in the summer. The owner was Bern Will Brown, a genuine northern eccentric who had been an oblate missionary. He had left that calling many years before and settled in this remote northern village.

Recently, he had married Margaret, a lovely younger woman of Inuit and European ancestry. His hobby was painting scenes of stereotypical northern life with Inuit and dog sled motifs. "These sell quite well," he told me.

Peggy and I opened our clinic in the cabin nursing station and started seeing the few patients that showed up. We slept in sleeping bags on bunk beds and kept the wood stove fire going. The next day we heard that Prince Charles and his party would not be coming for a few days since the airstrip was too soft and muddy, and unsafe for landing.

By then it was the weekend. We heard that the weather was improving, so we decided to wait. Peggy and I visited with the two RCMP officers brought over to Colville Lake to prepare the security of the town for the royal visit. By evening, Margaret came over to invite us for dinner.

After a fine dinner of caribou roast in the picturesque fishing lodge, Peggy said, "We have a special occasion today, it is Dr. Lacroix's birthday."

"Congratulations!" everybody answered.

Then, Bern Will got up and said, "I have something for you." He left the room for a few minutes and returned carrying a large thin parcel covered by an old blanket.

"This is a gift for you," he said.

I opened the blanket and found a large two foot diameter piece of gray shale, a flat rock containing a hand sized fossil of a double sea shell embedded in the middle. I gazed in amazement, as I was always fascinated by geology that explained the beginnings of our planet. This meant that this part of the continent had once been at the bottom of an ocean millions of years ago.

"Where did you find this?" I exclaimed.

"I found it near Lake DesBois," he said.

"Thank you. Thank you!" I answered gratefully.

Later, Peggy and I walked back to our cabin under the starry sky.

Two days later, the weather remained very sunny, but had cooled overnight so that the runway was judged hard enough to accept planes. We walked the short half-mile from the village to the airstrip, being careful not to leave the well-beaten path; if a person left the path, they would sink into the soft snow right up to their hips.

Thirty or so villagers stood with Peggy and I on one side of the runway. An RCMP officer stood in the middle of them, mingling discreetly with the crowd for security reasons. However he was a foot taller than the fairly short Dene native people, so his objective was impossible to fulfill. Security was not really a concern, though, as the local people were curious but reserved.

Finally a plane showed up, a Twin Otter, which is a twin-engine short takeoff and landing plane capable of carrying approximately 20 people. It landed with no incident on the slightly muddy landing strip. The plane was full of press people, who accompanied the royal tour everywhere.

Then the beautiful blue and white RCMP Twin Otter showed up and landed nicely, carrying the prince and his party. We stood in line wearing parkas and sunglasses against the sunny winter day, as Prince Charles shook each hand and said, "How do you do" to each person. As he was introduced to Peggy and me, his officials explained who we were. He asked a couple of short questions about what motivated us to come to such a remote place, then moved on. The meeting lasted perhaps 30 seconds.

His party and the planeload of press people almost outnumbered the local villagers. Then the prince and his party walked along the snowy path to the fishing lodge where a dog sled ride had been arranged for him, followed by refreshments.

Peggy and I started walking behind the entourage when a voice called, "Lianne is that you?"

I turned and a khaki parka clad man said, "Remember me? I am Pierre! I was in medical school a class ahead of you."

"Yes, of course I remember," I answered.

What a pleasant surprise. A colleague! After spending seven years in medical school, I certainly enjoyed meeting up with old friends. Pierre was an armed forces doctor now and had been assigned to accompany the prince on his Canadian tour.

The rest of the afternoon was most pleasant for me as I chatted with the friendly colleague from my own university in my own home city. Within an hour or two the visit was over and the whole group climbed onboard their two planes, safely taking off before the mud got too deep on the small runway.

Later that afternoon, a small plane landed on skies on the frozen lake, coming to take Peggy and I back to Fort Good Hope after our memorable days in Colville Lake. Carrying my large fossilized piece of rock, I returned to my small apartment in Inuvik, savoring the memories of my unusual experiences. The fossil traveled with me for the next 25 years living mainly in closets until I presented it to the Kelowna Museum where it now sits on permanent display.

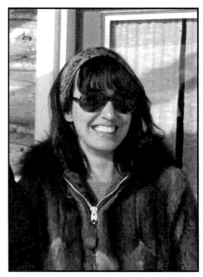

Winter sun in Colville Lake, April 1975.

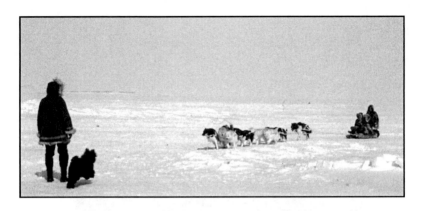

Prince Charles, Colville Lake toboggan ride and visit..

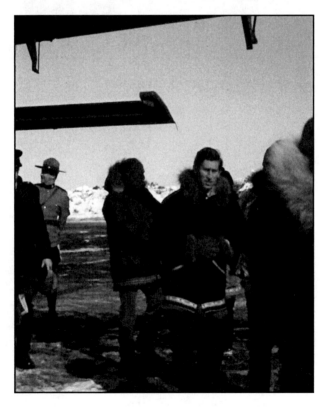

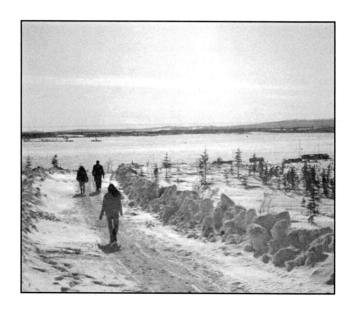

Colville Lake, April 1975.

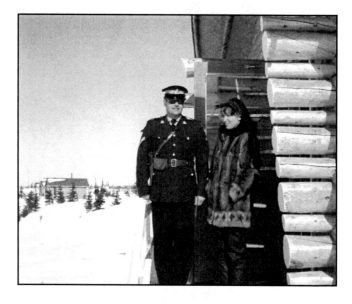

With RCMP officer in custom-made fur parka.

Box of Chocolates: 1975

It was a beautiful spring day with snow melting fast and mud holes appearing on our unpaved streets. I felt cheerful for no reason as I walked to the hospital.

As soon as I reached my desk, the phone rang. Chipo's voice said, "Dr Lacroix, we have one of your patients in early labour. Her name is Lois. I've checked her and she's 2 cm dilated."

My stomach tightened a bit. Lois was a petite delicate blond woman who had come to Inuvik from "down south" with her husband, Henry, an armed forces officer who was big-boned and around six feet tall. I was concerned that her baby would be too big for her small frame and that she would have complications. Our closest obstetrician was in Edmonton 1,300 miles away.

I walked to the case room and sat with Lois for awhile. She was indeed in good labour with contractions five minutes apart. She was breathing nicely with Henry as her coach. They had attended the popular local prenatal classes put on by our public health nurses.

I listened to the baby's heart with a fetoscope, similar to a stethoscope, but featuring a large round metal piece held on the mother's stomach. We had no electronic baby heart monitors of any kind at the time. On examining Lois, the baby was in the right position but seemed quite large.

As the day wore on, I went to see patients in the outpatient department and Lois carried on with her contractions that were now two minutes apart. Henry remained at her side helping in every way.

After several more hours we set up an IV to prevent dehydration. Every few hours I returned to check on her progress. Night came. We gave Lois a shot of Demerol and Gravol to get relief from the pain of her strong contractions while the labor continued. Epidurals were not available in small hospitals that did have a fully trained anesthetic specialist.

I went home and slept fitfully for a few hours. Myra, the night nurse called me several times to report on Lois' progress. There was little progress; she was only 4cm dilated. She had to become fully dilated to 10 cm, so that the baby would have enough room to pass through her cervix into this world.

Finally morning came. I got up, grabbed a peanut butter sandwich and walked fast to the hospital case room. Lois and Henry were both very tired while her labour continued as strong as ever. I examined Lois. She was still 4cm dilated, the baby was very big and the fetal heart was still good.

I said, "You have now been in good labour over 24 hours with no progress. The baby is too big for you. We'll have to do a Caesarian section… I'll call the surgeon."

Henry looked disappointed and Lois started to cry.

"You've done your best," I tried to reassure them. "The baby is still fine and we want a healthy baby and safe mother."

I paged Angelo and he came right away, as always. He listened to my history of the patient, and then went to talk to them. He examined the patient, which was the proper procedure.

"I agree," he said. "Lois needs a Caesarian section right away, before the other cases today."

We all went to the operating room where Angelo performed an efficient and rapid Caesarian section, with Lois under general anesthetic. She gave birth to a large 9lb baby boy in good condition.

Henry waited outside the surgical suite, as fathers were not allowed to attend emergency C-sections at the time.

When he first saw his baby he exclaimed, "It's Peter, I'd know him anywhere!" And he welcomed his son into the world.

We were all delighted as we wheeled the sleeping Lois to the Recovery Room. I felt greatly relieved that this story was ending well as obstetric complications are always possible. Lois recovered with no problems and went home in six days.

A week later a big box of chocolates arrived at our office addressed to Angelo and myself with a card that read, "With thanks, from Lois, Henry and Peter". We took the chocolates to the maternity ward for all to enjoy.

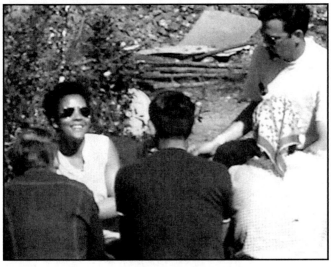

Nurse Chipo at a staff picnic.

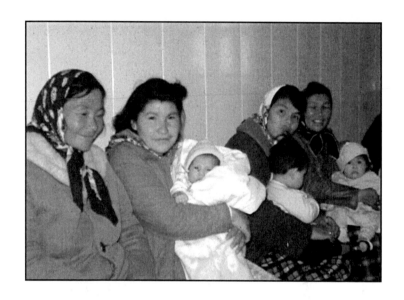

Clinic day.

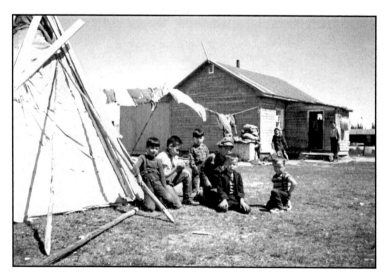

Boys at play.

FIVE

The Blue-Eyed Pilot: Spring 1975

March was always a difficult month in the arctic; the weather was still very cold and there were occasional snowstorms and white-outs, where land and sky blended into one big white fog.

Many of the hospital workers felt stressed or depressed and tempers would run short. We called it cabin fever; fatigue from unrelenting cold and darkness. My colleague Bill was the only one who seemed happy and oblivious to the weather; he had met his soul mate Shirley just a few months before.

Yet despite the winter gloom we also felt hope, as the hours of light slowly increased every day, chasing away the cobwebs.

It was time for me to return to Aklavik for my monthly visit. I caught a flight to carry me across the 40 miles that separated our towns.

After I had finished seeing the clinic patients, the nurse, Liz, said, "The zone director just called to say that he is coming over right away. He says that he wants to close the nursing station! He's chartered a plane and will be here within the hour."

The zone director was our supervisor, employed by Health and Welfare Canada to manage the staff of doctors and nurses who worked in our area.

We knew why he was coming. There had been a shooting in Aklavik a few days before, where one drunken man had killed another and had then been taken away by the local RCMP. The zone director was concerned about the safety of the nurses and for that reason he was talking about closing the nursing station.

The nurses and I were convinced that this shooting was an isolated incident. We did not want to close the station and leave the townspeople without medical care. The zone director arrived and after an hour of discussion we convinced him to see our point of view and to leave the nursing station open. We were very pleased and relieved.

Since the chartered plane was waiting to take the zone director back to Inuvik, I grabbed my bag and decided to catch the ride home. I walked from the large clinic room to the living room, where I found the pilot sitting on a couch trying to place some pieces of the puzzle that always rested on the small coffee table.

"Hi, I'm Ron," he said from across the room, too far to offer his hand.

"I'm Lianne," I answered. "We are ready to leave now."

We talked for a couple of minutes.

"I have a private pilot's licence," I told him.

By telling pilots this fact I hoped that they would let me sit with them in the front right seat which was much more interesting that the back seats. We walked over to the landing strip in front of the nursing station and boarded the Cessna 337, a light twin engine six person plane. The pilot did offer me the seat beside him. Nice guy, I thought. Nice blue eyes.

It was late evening, dark but clear as we flew over the frozen meandering channels of the Mackenzie River delta. Ron was very calm and obviously very competent and comfortable flying this plane back to Inuvik. We flew over the town in a big circle, slower than usual, marveling at the miniature buildings surrounded by dots of light in a white landscape. We landed on frozen Shell Lake, which served as the winter base of operations in Inuvik for Aklavik Flying Services, the local company that the hospital always hired. The zone director drove me back to town.

That pilot sure seemed nice, I thought to myself as we drove away. He's probably married, all the good ones are. And I never gave him another thought.

Six weeks later the receptionist at the hospital handed me a message.

It said, "Call Ron at this number." I walked to my apartment, thinking that there must be a form that I needed to sign from my last trip. I phoned the number. I barely remembered what Ron looked like.

A pleasant voice answered.

"No, it's not about a form," he said, "I just want to ask if you would like to go to dinner with me?"

That took me by surprise.

"Sure," I answered hopefully, "when did you have in mind?"

"How about Thursday?" he said, which was the next day. "We'll have dinner at the Eskimo Inn"

This was one of the two possible restaurants in town.

"Sure," I said.

We talked for perhaps another twenty minutes. He was very cheerful and lively and made me laugh, telling me that he was a very careful float plane pilot since he could not swim.

Thursday evening came. The doorbell rang and Ron walked into my apartment. He was slim with thick brown hair and lively blue eyes. He was very cheerful, chatty and outgoing. We drove in his car to the Eskimo Inn. It was May, 1975.

We looked at the menu, a little awkward with the newness of each other.

"I'll have the fish," I said to the waitress.

"We don't have any, sorry," she replied. "The plane did not bring supplies yesterday like we expected."

"I'll have the steak," said Ron.

"Sorry, not available either," said the waitress.

"How about a salad?" I countered

"Sorry, no," she replied.

"What do you have?" asked Ron finally.

She pointed to two items. So we ordered. Ron had the veal cutlets and I had the frog legs. Strange that these two items were available. It was the only time that I had ever had the opportunity to eat frog legs. They tasted like chicken.

We talked for a long time. It was easy. He was cheerful and we laughed a lot.

After dinner we walked across the muddy slippery unpaved road to his car. He took my hand and at that moment a strange new feeling came over me. I knew that this was *him*, that he was the one that I had been looking for, and that I had just met my life companion. It was a warm feeling in my heart and it felt strangely comfortable.

I do not necessarily believe that there is one special person for each of us; love has many seasons, it comes and goes for some and is hard to find for others.

I only know that for myself, in that moment, I looked at Ron's profile and thought, "He has a rather big nose but I know that this is the last time I will see him with my mind. Forever after I will look at him with my heart."

I expected that there would be difficulty ahead, as life is never smooth. But during that evening spent having dinner with the blue eyed pilot, I knew that my life had changed forever, that I had turned a corner and found the next path to follow.

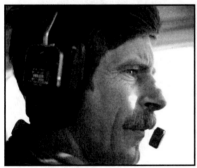

Ron, the pilot.

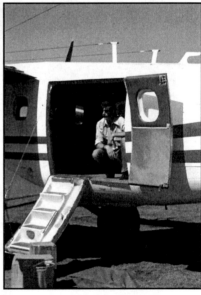

Ron in the doorway of a Twin Otter.

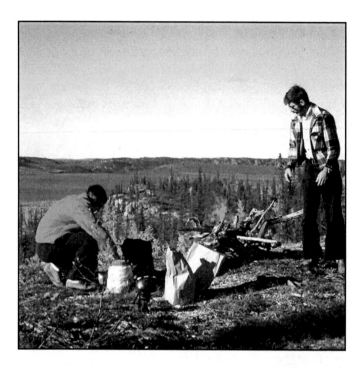

Picnic in the short arctic autumn.

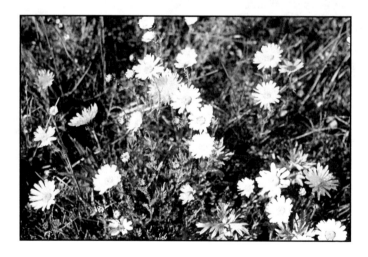

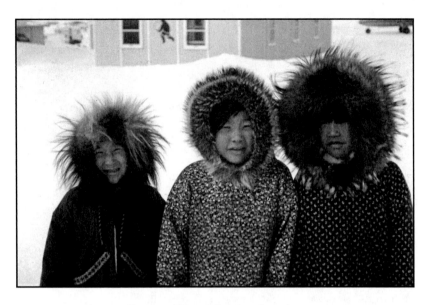

The people of Inuvik celebrating the winter games.

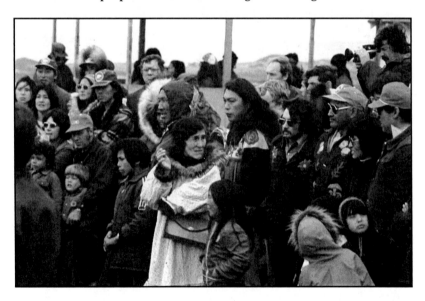

Knitted Red Socks: 1975

Every day, doctors who were not involved in assisting at surgery would see patients at the outpatient department, near the emergency room. Most patients made appointments and would choose to see the same doctor for their continuing medical care.

I was working there one day when the nurse said, "Dr. Lacroix there is a call for you from Iris, the nurse in Aklavik."

I answered right away.

The voice said, "Dr. Lacroix, this is Iris. I have a patient here that I am sending over. She's a 28 year old woman named Lucy who has severe abdominal pains and she is 4 months pregnant."

I remembered Lucy well. I had seen her at my previous visit and could not forget that she was pregnant and totally deaf. We could communicate with her only by writing. Some years before, she had been taught to write at a school down south. Communicating with her was quite slow as we wrote back and forth on a big sheet of paper.

She was a quiet, pleasant young Inuit native woman who lived with an older sister. The sister had told me that Lucy had a brief romance a few months before and that the boyfriend was long gone. The family had decided to give Lucy's baby to a married childless niece who would legally adopt the boy or girl. They felt that the child would have a more normal life this way.

Now I wondered whether she would have this child at all.

Within an hour Lucy arrived by stretcher and was admitted to our hospital. She was alone with no relatives. I took a history.

"Where does it hurt?" I wrote.

She pointed to her lower abdomen and wrote, "Here."

"How long?" I wrote.

"Two days," she wrote back in her large careful script.

I then examined her and found her lower abdomen tight and very tender. There was only one conclusion; she had an "acute abdomen".

We did a blood test which showed a normal white blood count, indicating that it was possibly not appendicitis. I was not sure. We had no ultrasound machines in those days as they were just becoming available in larger hospitals.

"I will call the specialist," I wrote to Lucy.

I paged Dr. DiStefano, who came to see her as soon as he finished his case in the operating room.

Angelo listened to my history of the patient, then patiently wrote questions to her. He was always very kind with sick people.

"We must operate right away," he said with no hesitation. "This woman has an acute abdomen, perhaps appendicitis or an ovarian cyst. This is not good for the pregnancy but we have no choice. If we do nothing, she will die," he added, and I knew that very well also.

We took Lucy to the OR and paged Bill to return and put her to sleep. After our usual scrubbing and gowning, Angelo opened her abdomen. I assisted and Sadie, the nurse, handed us the instruments.

We soon discovered that she had a large ovarian cyst the size of a grapefruit. It was called a chocolate cyst because of the colouring caused by old blood inside the liquid cyst. The cyst was not cancerous, but it was leaking and causing great pain.

Angelo easily and expertly removed the cyst and quickly closed her abdomen.

Within a week Lucy had recovered and took the plane back to her home in Aklavik.

Five months later Lucy returned to our hospital for her delivery. Since this was her first delivery, the nursing station in Aklavik could not keep her. They only kept low risk women who were delivering their second, third or fourth children. Women who had more than four children were called "grand multips" and because they faced other complications such as hemorrhaging, they could not be treated at nursing stations either.

I was called at three in the morning to attend the normal birth of her beautiful baby girl and Lucy did very well.

One month later as I was visiting Aklavik nursing station, Iris handed me a small package wrapped in brown paper. On the outside was written "From Lucy" in neat script. Inside was a pair of hand-knitted bright red socks with dark green toes and heels, a thank you from a grateful patient.

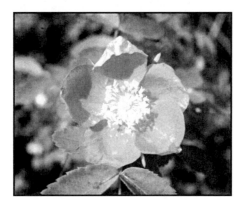

Fishing at Midnight: July 1975

Although we were always on call, we did not work all the time at our small arctic hospital. Sometimes we had an opportunity to do something fun and recreational.

One Friday evening, the phone rang in my apartment as Ron and I enjoyed one of our now-frequent visits.

"It's Tom," Ron stated.

Tom was Ron's best friend. He was another pilot, and his family owned Aklavik Air Services.

"He wants us to go fishing with him at a lake nearby," said Ron.

"When?" I asked.

"Right now!" he answered.

It was about eight in the evening. "Sure," I said.

We drove the few miles to Shell Lake where the float planes were located and climbed aboard a Cessna 185, a float plane that could hold 5-6 people. Our group was Ron and I, Tom, and two others. The small lake was calm like a mirror surrounded by spindly evergreen trees. Ron was piloting and the engine roared with power as it easily lifted into the calm evening; the sun was sinking into the western sky.

We flew north for about half an hour over low lying terrain covered by evergreens and thousands of small lakes of all shapes. Tom knew the country well. He had lived in Inuvik all his life; his father was one of the early bush pilots. The "Mike Zubko" Inuvik Airport bears his name.

Tom had been told by local Inuit that a certain unnamed lake was full of fish. Soon we were flying over this selected lake and, with calm expertise, Ron gently landed the plane, water splashing onto the floats. He headed towards the rocky shore. There was no sign of human life of any kind. It was a total wilderness.

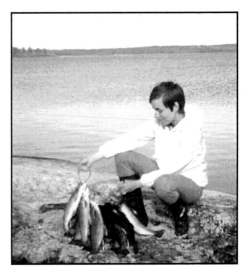

Arctic fish fry.

As the plane reached a narrow sandy beach between large rocks, Tom jumped out to shore and tied us to a large rock. I took out my tackle box. It had been some years since I had gone fishing, but I was keen to try again. Ron did not care for fishing so he started a small fire in case we caught something.

The sun was very low in the sky and we were fortunate to find few mosquitoes. I cast the first shot of my fishing rod and my line tangled and fell in the water only a few feet from shore, but to my surprise the line started moving and pulling. A fish was biting already! Quickly, I managed to get it ashore, and discovered it was a nice 2-3 pound arctic trout. Right away I caught another one and after a few minutes our group had caught several fish and cleaned them by the water's edge. We cooked our fish over the campfire and ate them by the light of the midnight sun. Then we removed all traces of our visit, pushed our floatplane back into the lake and flew home against the glowing pink sun, lying low in the northern sky.

Luck of the Draw: Old Crow, Fall 1975

Each doctor had a collection of remote villages which he visited monthly. If he moved away from Inuvik, the incoming doctor would inherit the assignment.

Maurice visited the towns of Norman Wells, Fort Norman and Fort Franklin. Ronald was assigned Fort Good Hope and Arctic Red River while Bill visited Tuktuyaktuk and Sachs Harbour to the north. The biggest settlement was my town, Aklavik, which was its own assignment as there were enough sick people there to occupy two or three days of clinic per month.

There was one special town, though, that was always reserved for the surgeon. While Old Crow barely contained two hundred people, it was considered big enough to have a nursing station. The surgeon would charter a plane for a one day visit, returning the same evening. We did not want to leave the hospital too long without surgical services in case there was some kind of emergency.

Old Crow was, in many ways, special. It was located below the tree line 200 miles due west of Inuvik in the Yukon Territory, and because most of the buildings were made of logs, it was quite picturesque. There was a strong community spirit; the people were Dene.

This was Angelo's village and our Italian surgeon grew very fond of his monthly trips there. Many times my boyfriend Ron flew him over early in the morning and waited for him to finish the clinic until they would fly home by late afternoon.

The lone nurse, Arlene, was always thrilled to see Angelo and would dress in her finest clothes the day that he visited.

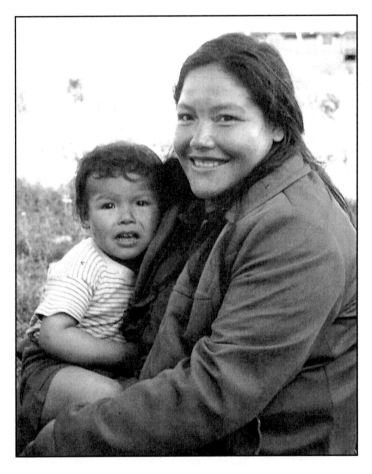

Native mother and child.

Angelo was very capable at practicing general medicine; he listened to the patients' chests and prescribed antibiotics which Arlene would dispense to the patient.

On one occasion Arlene said, "Dr DiStefano, this woman has been having abdominal pain for a long time," as she brought a middle aged woman into the clinic room.

Angelo examined her and Arlene checked her hemoglobin on the little portable machine. This was the only test available.

"We need to send this lady to the hospital but not urgent," said Angelo, "I suspect gallstones and we should remove them."

Arlene explained this diagnosis to the patient, who wanted to talk to her family before going to the hospital the following week.

At noon Angelo, Arlene and the pilot would have lunch with the finest foods that could be found in her nursing station pantry, prepared by Bertha, the local domestic helper. Then they would see a few more patients and Angelo would fly home late in the day, hoping that no surgical emergency awaited his return to the hospital.

This man, who came from a very sunny, very civilized and ancient country far away, had nicely adapted to the magnificent, cold, raw land sparsely populated by an endearing people. Angelo was given several presents by people who were grateful for his services. He proudly wore a pair of caribou hide mittens decorated with brightly coloured beaded designs made by the local ladies from his town.

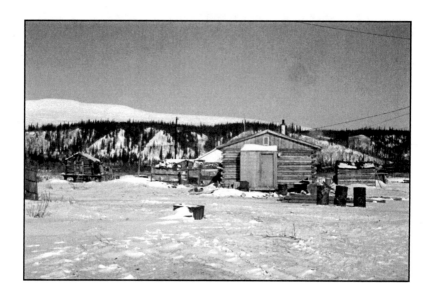

Old Crow, Angelo's village.

Angelo's Romance: Summer 1975

One summer evening in 1975, the medical staff all gathered on the steps of the hospital and we had our portrait taken. Bill had met Shirley, I had met Ron and our smiles reflect our happiness.

A few weeks later, a new operating room nurse called Barbara arrived at our hospital. She came from Toronto and lived in the nurses' residence with about thirty colleagues. She was in her mid-twenties, a beautiful natural blonde woman whose beauty was as evident on her inside as on her outside. She met Angelo at work as the surgical assisting nurse on his various surgeries. She soon became Angelo's constant companion and we could see them walking downtown together. They had a special connection and within a few weeks Barbara moved into his town house. The two of them seemed very happy together.

A couple of months later, as the land was suddenly reclaimed by the implacable cold and darkness of winter, we heard the strange news that Angelo's wife and daughter from Italy were coming for a visit. Angelo had always told us that he and his wife had been separated for many years, since he left Rome to study in the US, while his wife and daughter stayed in Italy. We were surprised by this turn of events.

Barbara quickly moved back to the nurses' residence.

We did not see much of Angelo for the next two weeks nor did we get to meet his family. He was more quiet than usual. He just did his hospital work then went straight home.

I phoned him once during this time regarding a patient and I could hear the unhappiness in his voice as we talked. Perhaps they were discussing their divorce, I thought, but did not ask. Then Stella and the daughter were gone.

A week or two later Barbara and Angelo resumed their happy life together and we all continued our medical work to help the local population. Our snowy dark arctic world seemed very far away from historic sunny Italy.

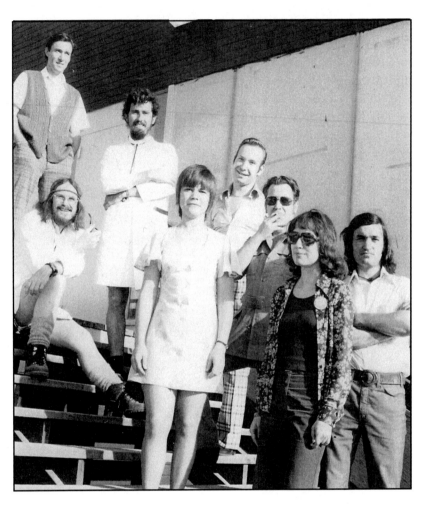

Medical staff at Inuvik General Hospital, summer 1975.
Clockwise: Bill Sara (sitting), Frank Kelly, Stuart McDonald, Corrine
Stewart (medical secretary), Rene Turnow (dentist), Angelo DiStefano,
Lianne Lacroix, Ronald Calderisi.

Double Turkeys: December 1975

Over two years had passed since I had come to Inuvik and Christmas rolled around again. I was now engaged to Ron and living in a pastel colored two storey townhouse two blocks from the hospital. Many of our friends like Angelo and Ronald were away for Christmas or doing something else

At Christmas time that year, Bill and Shirley decided to elope. Since they had so many friends in town and did not want a big fussy wedding, they decided to fly to Sachs Harbour, the remote village that Bill visited each month. In the darkness of winter they were married by a Justice of the Peace in a private ceremony witnessed by a handful of their relatives. It was a fitting arctic wedding for a man who belonged to that land so well. This was his farewell tour of the high arctic since they had decided to move to the mountains near Calgary, Alberta. I said goodbye to my old friend; our work lives had been closely connected for over two years.

In the meantime Ron and I were planning to enjoy our first Christmas together in the arctic, just the two of us with a small turkey. Two weeks previously, I had bought one at the local Hudson's Bay store and since our fridge was quite small, we decided to keep it in the trunk of Ron's car; the temperature there remained steady around 40° below zero. There was no chance that it would melt.

Three days before Christmas, I removed the plastic of the turkey and wrapped it in brown paper. Then I placed it in the refrigerator which, according to my Betty Crocker cookbook, would sufficiently defrost it prior to cooking. Christmas morning came but the turkey was still frozen hard. Indeed the whole fridge seemed much colder than usual. There was no way to cook that bird. Then it dawned on us! The turkey's temperature was down to 40° below zero in that car trunk. The fridge hovers around freezing. The turkey had cooled the fridge, but had not warmed itself at all.

"What to do, what to do?" I said.

The phone rang. Ron answered.

"It's Tom," he said "Wishing us compliments of the season."

Tom was to be the best man at our wedding. Ron explained our problem to him.

Then Ron turned around and said, "Tom is asking us to come over. He has one of those new microwave ovens and says that maybe it could defrost our turkey."

We drove over to the Tom and Andrea's, put the turkey in the microwave and tried melting it. No luck, the skin melted a bit and the bird scorched perhaps an inch deep, but nothing else.

Andrea asked us to stay, so we spent the Christmas dinner at Tom and Andrea's eating their turkey.

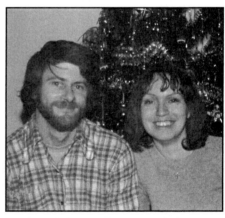

By Boxing Day our turkey was finally defrosted enough that Ron and I could cook it. We invited Tom and Andrea to our place to eat that arctic turkey and thus the two couples spent Christmas together with double turkeys.

First Christmas for Ron and Lianne.

A Thousand Lindas: 1976

The days of the winter followed one another, busy as always. Ron was flying people across the arctic while I was working hard at the hospital, on call most of the time. I felt happy and cheerful now that I had found my partner; we enjoyed our time together.

One day as I was seeing patients at the hospital's outpatient department, the nurse Penny said, "The next patient is a young girl named Linda who is here for a pregnancy test. The lab is doing it now."

We had a new twenty minute urine pregnancy test which was a big improvement over the earlier two hour version.

"I'll put the patient in the room," said Penny, "Here are the results."

I walked into the exam room. Linda was a pretty 16 year old Métis girl of Dene and European ancestry. I remembered seeing her picture in "The Drum", our local newspaper, as she had graduated from grade ten a few months earlier, winning many awards.

She sat quietly looking at the floor.

"We have your pregnancy test and it's positive," I said gently. "This means that you are pregnant."

She immediately burst into loud tears. I grabbed my ever present box of Kleenex and moved it closer to her.

"Not good news, is it?" I asked quietly.

When she calmed down, Linda said, "I knew it. I missed my period and I was not feeling well. I don't want to be pregnant. I don't want to quit school. I want to be a lawyer. I can't have a baby!" Then she cried some more.

"Doctor, you've got to help me," she said, sobbing again.

"What about your boyfriend?" I asked gently. "How does he feel about this?"

"I don't have a boyfriend," she sobbed, "I went to a party, had some drinks, don't remember much…" her voice trailed off.

"What about your parents?" I asked.

"I just have my Mom," said Linda. "She'll help me, I've already told her everything. I want to go for… an operation…"

We talked a few more minutes discussing her options. Linda was determined. She had made her decision. She wanted an abortion.

"I'll phone the specialist and let you know," I answered as she left.

At the time abortions were legal in this country and available in big cities like Edmonton. The family doctor had to make the referral to the specialist and write a letter of support. Then the case was reviewed by a hospital committee before approval.

As I sat at the desk writing in her file, I well remembered the one occasion, during my final year of medical school, when I had witnessed a therapeutic abortion. The gynecological specialist had said to me, "The next one is yours," meaning that I could do the next procedure.

"No, I can't do it," I answered, "because of my religion."

I had been brought up in a strict Roman Catholic family where abortion was a sin and condemned at every opportunity. It felt wrong to me and I could not do it.

However the religion of my family was also very personal. We did not explain our beliefs to anyone and we did not try to convert anyone. We respected other people and their beliefs.

Something in the young girl's distress had touched my heart. It did not seem fair that a two minute mistake would change her life forever while the young man involved suffered no consequence whatsoever. I knew I needed to help her, but whom could I talk to? I had not discussed this issue with my male colleagues and felt that the burden did not need to be shared with the young male doctors. I knew that Angelo was likely Catholic, so it never crossed my mind to ask him to perform the operation.

I felt that it was not up to me to tell people what to do. I really believe in the right of women to make their own choices in life. I respect the doctors who choose to perform abortions; it is their decision. I respect the doctors who are against abortions, as that is their choice as long as they provide the correct information to their patients.

My own course of action was chosen after careful reflection. I chose to help by providing a referral, and then I silently vowed that in my medical career I would work to prevent such heart breaking situations.

I walked to our phone and called the specialist in Edmonton. As I waited for the long distance operator to connect me, a memory surfaced in my mind of another Linda - I'll call her by that name, who had died some fifteen years before.

While I was a laboratory tech student, the autopsy and pathology departments were situated on the same floor as our laboratories. Every so often we would see orderlies pushing stretchers of deceased people covered by white sheets.

One day as I left for coffee, the utility elevator door opened and another sheet-covered body wheeled past me. When I returned fifteen minutes later a hush had fallen over the usually cheerful lab workers.

"Why is everybody so quiet?" I asked the lab tech beside me at our counter.

"We hear that the body that went past is that of an 18 year old girl who has died from a backstreet abortion," she whispered.

This was in the early 1960's, when abortions were still illegal in Canada.

I was horrified. She was my exact age. She had made a mistake. She was looking for romance and love and had found despair and death! It was not fair!

The man involved suffered nothing and perhaps he did not even know. I was outraged. I tried my best to put the incident out of my mind, until now...

"Hello, switchboard," said a voice far away from the Edmonton hospital.

"May I speak with the gynecologist on call?" I asked, as my mind returned to this Linda.

I explained the situation to him and he agreed to see my patient for the procedure. I wrote a letter on her behalf saying that she needed the surgery to preserve her physical and mental health.

Linda and her mother left for Edmonton the next day. I spent the day sitting in my office dictating files, thinking that there must be a better way of preventing such situations.

A few years later I joined Planned Parenthood (now called Options for Sexual Health), where I would work for many decades with the goal of helping other Lindas *before* they used up half a box of Kleenex during an unexpected visit to the doctor's office.

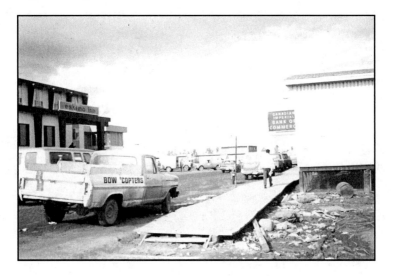

Raised boardwalks in Inuvik in the summer.

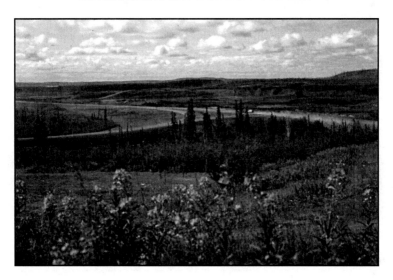

The vast expanse of land and sky near Inuvik.

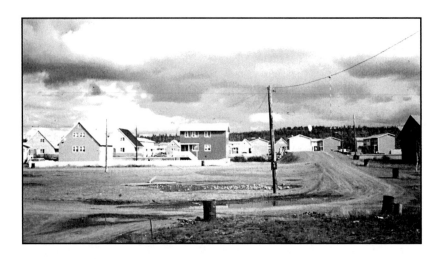

Inuvik street scene in the summer.

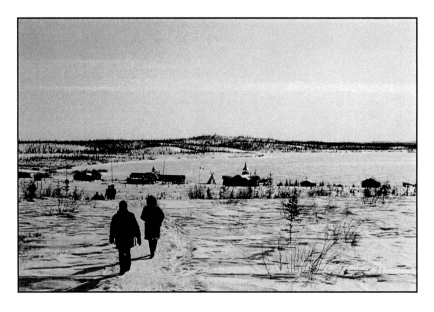

Springtime in Colville Lake.

SIX

Our Impostor Surgeon: February 1976

It snowed for several days but just small amounts. The snow was never very deep in Inuvik, perhaps because the 40° below zero temperature kept moisture away from our region. As February crept along, the sun provided more and more light every day.

One Saturday morning the phone rang.

"Hello?" I answered.

The voice was familiar and anxious.

"Hi, it's Barb, Angelo's been arrested by the police! They say there's a problem with his papers ...that he's an impostor! I don't know what to do."

I was speechless for a few seconds!

"How did this happen?" I asked.

"We don't know anything at this point," she said. "I just needed to phone and tell you. I can't imagine that there is any truth to it, can you?"

"Angelo's a terrific surgeon, Barb, we all know that. Please keep us posted and let us know if there is anything that we can do," I answered, and hung up the phone in a state of shock.

An impostor is someone who passes himself off as being qualified in a profession when in fact he is not, I said to myself, trying to grasp the meaning of these events.

There was no question of Angelo DiStefano's surgical skills in my mind. I had worked closely with him for about a year and a half and this news made no sense at all...I was stunned....I did not believe it! There must be some mistake; Angelo was the best surgeon we had seen during my years in Inuvik.

A few hours later, my fiancé Ron returned from a flight and was equally distressed about the news.

"They think that Angelo is a fake?" he exclaimed. "I don't believe it for one second!"

Angelo always requested Ron as his pilot when he visited Old Crow and they had shared many pleasant and lengthy conversations. Ron felt that he knew Angelo quite well, and did not have any doubts about him.

"Not everybody likes Angelo, maybe, but he's obviously a qualified and proficient surgeon!" Ron answered. His track record proved his ability; how could a person perform complex surgeries, successfully, if he wasn't a trained surgeon? It seemed preposterous.

We learned that Angelo was being held by the local RCMP detachment for questioning for the next three days and that he was allowed to see only Barbara, and only for a few minutes each day.

Barb was in touch with us daily. She told us that Angelo was very upset, and could not sleep or eat. At her insistence, Ronald and Maurice were allowed to see him on the third day. I was busy at the hospital with a lady in labour and could not accompany them.

Finally Angelo was released and went back to his home with Barbara to await further developments. He was warned not to leave town and told that he would have to appear before a judge in Yellowknife by the end of that week.

The press came to talk to Maurice, who had been named Chief of Staff after Bill and Shirley moved to Alberta two months before. They asked him for a statement and he was quoted as saying, "Dr. DiStefano has worked with us for almost 18 months and provided exemplary medical services to the patients of this hospital."

At the hospital, all booked surgeries were cancelled and urgent cases were sent by plane to Edmonton. All of the hospital staff was stunned that our surgeon had been arrested as an impostor and a quiet gloom settled over our usually cheerful workplace.

Globe and Mail Newspaper: February 20, 1976

'Above-average surgeon performed 350 operations: Doctor accused of forgery saved lives, co-workers say"

Special to the Globe and Mail

YELLOWKNIFE--The man wanted in Italy for forgery and posing as a doctor saved many lives in the Inuvik General Hospital operating room, according to his professional colleagues.

Dr. Angelo Di Stefano, chief of surgery, was granted conditional bail yesterday following his arrest last week on charges laid under the Immigration and Extradition Acts.

The immigration charge said he used false information to

enter Canada in 1974. The Extradition Act charges say he is wanted in Italy on fraud and misrepresentation charges laid in 1971. The warrant for his arrest alleges the 40 year old Italian immigrant also goes under the aliases of Aldo Alessiani, Ivan Stefanovic and Angelo diSterfano.

But in Inuvik, the doctor who assisted the Italian at more than 350 operations calls him "an above-average surgeon and an extraordinary man."

"I am most impressed by his clinical judgment and bedside diagnosis," said Dr. Ron Calderisi in a long-distance interview from the Inuvik hospital.

"There are several people who owe their lives to him."

Dr. Calderisi's sentiment was echoed by the hospital's chief of staff, Dr. Maurice E. Myers.

Dr. Calderisi assisted Dr. DiStefano, who he says is his closest friend, at an emergency operation last October on a 4 year old child who was accidentally shot in the chest by her brother. "He certainly saved her life and she's in excellent shape," Dr. Calderisi said.

The surgeon is also credited with expert handling of two critical cases last month. He operated successfully on a man stabbed in the heart and the gastric artery, and he repaired the kidney and grafted the iliac artery on a man crushed by a snowmobile.

"It was no orderly that did that." agreed Dr. Di Stefano's girlfriend, nurse Barbara Mills, who flew down from Inuvik to be in the courtroom yesterday.

The pretty blonde, who quit her job as intensive care nurse in

Toronto General Hospital, looking for "challenge and excitement in the arctic," said she met the doctor when she arrived in Inuvik five months ago.

"He's very skilled and I have the utmost admiration for Angelo, even if I weren't personally involved with him."

She complained that he was kept for three days in a small dark jail cell in Inuvik where he was deprived of cigarettes and allowed to see visitors for only five minutes a day. "The RCMP treated him like a murderer."

The bail hearing was complicated because the man is wanted by another country. The news media were banned from reporting any of the proceedings, which included details of the man's personal and professional background.

Bail was granted by Mr. Justice William Morrow of the N.W.T. Supreme Court under several strict provisions including the condition the man leave his bank account and passport in the hands of the Mounties, who will let him have $50 a day for expenses.

He will spend each night in jail and must report to the RCMP twice each day. Bail ends March 1, by which time Italian authorities are likely to arrive in Inuvik to return him to Italy to face charges. The doctor was barred this week from practicing medicine by the N.W.T. Government pending an investigation.

Dr. Calderisi said his friend's problems stem from his involvement as a left-wing political activist during his student days in Italy in the late 1950's.

"I knew about some of his past. But there were some things he had kept to himself." the family practitioner said. "I told him about a month ago he has a story that should be told. His father was a magistrate in Rome, who wanted Angelo to be a magistrate. But he wanted to be a doctor."

"He used to shine shoes in the Roman train station to get enough money to buy a microscope in first year medical school." The two doctors met for the first time in Inuvik 15 months ago.

Dr. DiStefano was slated to fly back to Inuvik in the RCMP plane last night. The RCMP offered Miss Mills a seat in the plane for the return flight.

Action on the Immigration Act charge was stayed until March 1 to give Dr. DiStefano an opportunity to return to Italy under the extradition proceedings.

Angelo's Inuvik Farewell: February 28, 1976

The people of the town were also upset over this turn of events. They did not believe that there could be anything wrong with Angelo as he had literally saved many of their lives or the lives of their loved ones. Our local newspaper weighed in on the story, though it seemed to us that they went out of their way to make Angelo seem incompetent; sensational stories are more interesting whether true or not.

Ron and I met with Angelo for coffee at his house a few days after he returned from Yellowknife. He was busily packing and gave me his espresso maker, which I never used, since specialty coffees were unknown to us in the 1970's.

We learned that he had been granted bail while the authorities arranged for his extradition to Italy. We saw the stress on his face but he seemed quietly determined to go and answer to the charges, whatever they may be, in the sunny country of his birth.

A few days later, I saw Angelo in our common office in the hospital, finishing up the dictating of his last patient files. It would be the last time I saw him.

"I want you to know the truth about me," he said in French, and he handed me a collection of legal sized typed pages.

I looked at the package, then at him, and he said, "I have written it all down and explained everything."

Angelo had dictated the complete explanation of his story into our hospital dictation system. Our medical secretary, Corrine, typed them up and photocopied them for his closest friends.

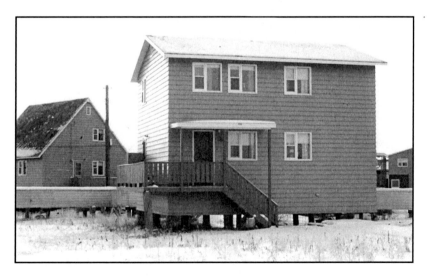

Angelo DiStefano's residence in Inuvik.

Lianne Lacroix

We hugged briefly, then he was gone.

 Even then we both knew it was unlikely that he would ever return to Inuvik but we promised to keep in touch by letter and meet again some day.

I watched him walk away wearing his heavy parka and embroidered mittens, and felt that a golden age of medicine at Inuvik General Hospital was suddenly coming to a close. We would never see again such a wonderful competent colourful surgeon; an era was closing and I felt sad to see him leave under a dark cloud of suspicion.

The next day at the hospital, rumors started flying around as several personnel expressed doubts – now that Angelo was gone. Details and events were reviewed and discussed. Because such little information was available about what was happening, suspicion floated down the halls of our familiar building. Even Maurice seemed to wonder if he had done the right thing by defending Angelo's work. Doubt is a very damaging and insidious disease.

"I knew there was something different about him," said Larry, the doctor who had never liked Angelo in the first place.

"He's a lot older that he claims," our hospital dentist, Neil, stated as he stood in the cafeteria lineup. "I looked at his teeth you know. You can tell a lot from a person's teeth."

It was strange and disturbing to see how some remained true committed friends while others wavered and crossed over to the doubting side...

Our colleague Ronald was especially upset. Angelo was his closest friend and he did not take kindly to the 'Doubting Thomases' of the hospital. Like my fiancé Ron and I, he defended Angelo at every conversation. Indeed after discussing his options with his fiancée, Diane, they decided to leave Inuvik within the month. Ronald was too upset to stay without his friend and mentor and returned south where he started training to become a surgeon himself.

I read Angelo's confession but did not show it to anyone outside our circle of close friends. I felt that some of the other coworkers might very well interpret the confession differently, and did not want to give them more fodder.

I learned that Angelo had been a Communist but it made no difference to me as I knew that in Italy, the Communists were a political party; people in that country were often Catholic and Communist together. I had no doubts because I had seen this man's noble side on a daily basis; his competence and his sympathy for our patients were all that mattered

Barbara was devastated and took a leave of absence from her nursing duties for two weeks so that she could absorb what was happening to her life. She returned to her work at the hospital while Angelo's court case was underway in Italy. After two months she returned to her home town in Ontario as Angelo's case seemed to be resolving. She considered herself engaged to Angelo and looked forward to joining him somewhere to start their life together. Ron and I said goodbye to her knowing that we would likely never meet again…

We would learn of the couple's fate through a series of letters sent to us from Italy.

Angelo's Confession
Dated: February 28, 1976 Inuvik N.W.T.

Dictated through the Hospital Dictaphone[1]:

I am Dr. Angelo DiStefano. Today is Saturday the 28th of February 1976. I have only 16 hours left before I surrender myself for extradition purposes to return to Italy and face my charges. The reason I refused all press interviews, the only reason, is that the RCMP warned me to be careful what I said to the press.

On the 13th of February at 9pm an RCMP constable and sergeant arrived at my home in Inuvik. They did not arrest me. They said there was some irregularity about my papers and they wanted to see me in their office. I was already in bed. I dressed myself. I prepared myself and went to their office with hope and said to my girlfriend---I consider her my wife and I hope that we will be married as soon as possible --- not to worry, that I would come back soon because my conscience is clear.

They questioned me all night. They charged me that my papers were forged; they charged me for many things. I will now tell you the other side.

The next day, Saturday, they started again, and Sunday; they questioned me all weekend. They allowed me to see my girlfriend Barbara for five or ten minutes a day. I became very depressed and humiliated and I could not eat even the grapes and milk that Barbara brought me.

One night they brought me to Yellowknife (capital of N.W.T. 700 miles away by plane) I went through the bail for

---

[1] Author's comments appear in italics.

extradition and for the Immigration Act. They fought really hard not to give me bail. Finally Mr. Justice Morrow gave me very strict bail. I must return twice a day at 2pm and 7pm and come to sleep in the cell from 11pm to 11am the next day for 10 days. I am taping this on the 9th day of my partial freedom. I wish to thank Judge Morrow that he gave me this opportunity...I have some previous commitments to my girlfriend to explain what happened because she does not know anything. I never told her anything before and he gave me the opportunity to spend some time with her before going to Italy. I hope to marry her some day and to have a family like every happy family in the world, a family based on work and honesty and love.

I worked until a few days ago when I resigned, I worked for National Health and Welfare as a surgeon in this zone. Well I worked with all my heart for 16 months. I dedicated myself for 24 hours a day for Canada and before this happened, I was an integral part of the system of this country.

Next week I will return to Rome. I surrendered myself as I said before and hope to get faster justice in Rome. The Rome extradition talks about forgery of medical documents which is not true. This forgery in Rome was supposed to have been committed in Rome between February and April 1971. I have evidence that this is not true because my passport is stamped showing that I was in Rhodesia during this time. How is it possible to be in Rhodesia and commit a crime in Italy?

The real reason that Italy wants me, that they want to prosecute and judge me, is for my political beliefs and for instigating demonstrations. I am a Communist. I *was* a Communist, because I resigned last January and gave up completely the Italian Communist Party. I fell in love with this girl Barbara who changed completely my beliefs of 23 years.

How I became a Communist, I remember that. I was thirteen years old in 1947-48 and Italy was very hungry. The whole population was very hungry. (*This was post WWll when Italy had been under the control of Fascist dictator Mussolini who had taken the side of Hitler and the Nazis. They were defeated by the Americans who occupied the country*). I went to the garbage of the Americans who occupied the country to find something to eat. One Negro soldier he beat me up only for looking in the garbage. From this moment I started to hate everything that was imperialist, everything that was rich people against the poor people.

I was interested right away by the Italian Communist Party at 18 years old when I started my first year of University. (*Communists teach that all are equal and wealth should be divided among all workers*).

I am a doctor! I did my six years of university 1953-1959....I came from a good wealthy family, the Marquis family of Serracapriola *(southern Italy)*. My father was a magistrate and when he died in 1974, he was Chief Justice of Italy. He was against me for becoming a doctor but mostly because I was a Communist. He pulled me out of my home and threw me out. He did not want to hear anything more from me. I was 18 years old. I gave my application to the university medical school and I did so many things, *(to support himself)*. I was a doorman in a nightclub, a waiter, and cleaned shoes to pay my fees for university.

Now, in this period we began to organize demonstrations against the government. I remember in 1952-to--54 when Eisenhower came to Rome, when many political people in the United States came to Rome, I was the one who organized many demonstrations against these people.

In 1959 the police killed two of our people in the university, two students at the university. To demonstrate against these two killings we burned the University of Rome. This was June 1959. I was ready to take my thesis.

I prepared my thesis with Professor Bosco. After the police took us out of the university, the president of the University of Rome and the Minister of Public Education of Rome expelled me from all universities in Italy and denied me from doing my thesis.

It was at this time that I came to the United States. I was still always affiliated with the Italian Communist Party. I came to the Detroit General Hospital and did my five years of residency in surgery. I stopped one time for one year, around 8 or 9 months because any place that needed help, I was there. I was in France in 1961-62 when the Algerians were fighting for their freedom. The Italian Communist party and the French Communist party were trying to help the Algerians.

Today the Detroit General denies that I was there because I did not have permanent residence with Immigration and if they admit it, they must pay a $100,000 fine to Immigration. The Detroit General knew very well that I only had a tourist visa, but they needed residents (*doctors training to become specialists*) very badly. The doctors in America are very busy in private practices and no one would do the residency, only foreigners. I remember that I was the only Italian among 32 Cuban doctors---that's where I learned my Spanish. I didn't learn my English there. I learned Spanish at this time in the nine years that I was there. They knew very well that I had a tourist visa but today, today they deny that I was there.

Even Dr. Cantor denies it. I worked nine years with him. I worked with Professor Plauss, Professor Friedman...I remember well, because he died in the OR during a caesarean section. I was his first assistant when he died of a heart attack. There are traces of this in the old records. In 1966 I was Chief Resident of the Detroit General. Professor Cantor and I started my pathology *(training)* over there. Well all these things they deny today.

But I don't care because my conscience is clear. My only crime is a belief ...what I believed when I became a doctor and before I became a doctor...that I must help people who are suffering not only physically by some sickness or disease but to help people who are oppressed.

It is the reason that I went to Rhodesia in 1971 to help these people. I helped organize demonstrations. One of them turned into a riot in Fort Victoria in 1972. This was not successful for the oppressed black people. However the voice of freedom of these people was heard around the world and every part of the world heard the cry of these black people suffering in their own land. For trying to help poor people I am suffering today for my beliefs.

For these beliefs I will be suffering and going by handcuffs to Italy to trial, separated from the one I love. I never in my life stole one cent, one simple cent from anyone. I gave away all my money. Today I am poor. I must borrow some money from my girlfriend if I want to pay for some help in Rome. I never killed anybody. I never stole from anybody. I never took any property from anybody.

Here in Inuvik, I invite you people to talk to any doctor at this hospital and the whole population Eskimo and Indian from Tuktoyaktuk to Sachs Harbor or Paulatuk, any place. Ask them how many lives I have saved. It is not my duty to tell myself how many lives, the medical records and my colleagues in Inuvik will tell you how much good I did and how many lives I saved...It is not for me to tell that.

The police have charged that I have no Fellowship in Surgery in my papers. I must clarify that I did the F.A.C.S. *(exams to become a specialist)* and I did that in Chicago in 1965 and after the Fellowship of the American College of Surgeons found out that I didn't have the final thesis in Rome...I passed my examinations and I invite you people to go to Chicago and check, for in July 1965, I wrote my full examinations. That is what is recorded in Glasgow (Scotland) in 1974.

When I came to Canada, I came with a contract written by the provincial government signed by Dr. Collingwood who employed me. I was at St. John's Memorial University with Professor Campbell in pathology. I was teaching and went two times a week to Placentia Bay to operate. I have a full licence in Newfoundland which I renewed...I have here the proof and the evidence, the last $50 cheque I sent for 1976.

The reason that I came to Inuvik follows. The Immigration and Manpower Department convoked me and said that if I wanted to become a landed immigrant without leaving Canada, with the new law, I must go to Inuvik to help *(an underserviced area)*. Then I would become a landed immigrant in a reasonable length of time without leaving the country.

That is the way I accepted to come to Inuvik on salary. I did not come here to open a private practice to make money..no...one poor salary to work 24 hours a day for 365 days a year. I am here for 16 months.

On the 16 of January 1976, Immigration Canada gave me my landed immigrant status with the remark "for national interest". I invite you people to check this out. I showed these papers to my friends at the hospital. I have to tell you that last September 11, 1975, the ambassador of Italy was here in Inuvik. He was a guest at my house. I met him at the Eskimo Inn with a group of officials from Ottawa who came to the north for the pipeline *(natural gas pipeline planning to be built)*. The ambassador was here. I correspond almost weekly with the Italian Embassy. I was not hiding myself. All the Italian authorities know where I am. The President of the Italian

Republic sent me congratulations for being the only surgeon above the Arctic Circle. The copy of this letter was given by my girlfriend to the Toronto Star reporter and the original went to my lawyer in Italy.

I am finished with this little story. Next week I will be out of Canada. I helped the natives. All the natives in the Inuvik district are with me. Everybody has sent letters to the priest to pray for me and they are doing all possible for me but I am leaving Canada. I am leaving with my heart broken. I am only a man who came here to help the people but I must leave in handcuffs without any big reason. My heart is broken.

Well, I must leave with the hope of returning as soon as possible to marry my love. I must come back because my only reason for living is my girlfriend that I want to marry as soon as I get my divorce in Italy. I want to live in peace with my girlfriend. My home is Canada. My conscience is very clear. Everything in me is clear and I will face every charge.

Thank you for listening to me. I swear on the Bible and I swear to God that every word said on this tape is true, wholly true. Everything is true, dictated from my heart, this broken heart of one man...40 years old...who for 23 years has only followed his beliefs... Thank you for listening to me............

Letter from Dr. Ronald Calderisi to the People of Fort Good Hope: 1976

I will be holding my last clinic in Fort Good Hope on March 30-31. It has been an honor, privilege and pleasure serving as your settlement doctor for the past 18 months and I feel that I will be leaving friends.

The reason for my sudden decision to leave government service is my disenchantment and profound disappointment with the manner in which my closest and most trusted friend Dr. Angelo DiStefano, has been treated by Canadian authorities.

Dr. DiStefano is an above average surgeon with outstanding skills and is an extraordinary, intense and courageous man. He has saved many lives and improved the quality of many others.

Dr. DiStefano's medical training and surgical abilities are beyond reproach. I would want him to operate on me or my mother or father if an operation was necessary.

In his final year of medical school in Rome, he was expelled from university because he had organized a student demonstration protesting the murder of two students by fascist police. He has been a very active freedom fighter throughout his professional career. He was sentenced to death twice, once in France for assisting Algerians in their fight for independence and once in Rhodesia for aiding black nationalists in their fight for freedom in their own land.

His only crime is that he is a Marxist, believing in world socialism and freedom for all. When he went to Detroit in 1959 to study surgery, American Immigration officials continuously refused to grant him a working visa because of his political beliefs. He spent at least five years in Detroit studying surgery and pathology but the Detroit Hospital denies it today, to avoid a $100,000 fine for employing a man without a working visa.

These are some of the many facts that will come out in greater detail later. Enough said as I am leaving the employment of this government in protest.

I love the North too much not to return. If the Dene ever realize their dream of an independent nation I would love to return and work for you.

Kindest regards, Ron Calderisi MD

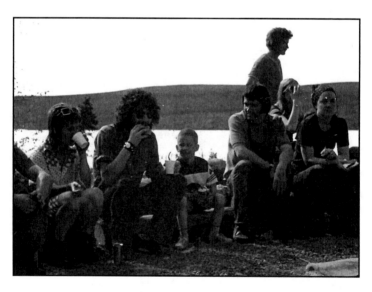

The good days: a staff picnic during the brief arctic summer.

SEVEN

Hospital in the Spring: 1976

The days followed one another, busy and active in the spring of 1976. The snow was finally melting and the townspeople were placing bets as to the exact date of *breakup*, the day that the waters of the Mackenzie River would again flow freely thanks to the breakup of the ice pack.

Dr. Scott, a surgeon from Edmonton, had been sent by Health and Welfare to review Angelo's patient files. Patient charts were always up to date and totally legible as our files were all dictated and then typed by our medical secretary, Corrine.

At the end of the week we asked Dr. Scott if he found anything to criticize in Angelo's charts.

Quietly, Dr. Scott answered, "He performed a lot of surgeries from a wide variety of specialties, which is unusual, but everything seems to be in order." That was the last we heard of the matter of Angelo's surgical performance.

A new surgeon arrived at our hospital. John was young and was literally a *new* surgeon. He was a very caring and keen doctor, but he just did not have the wide experience and advanced training that Angelo had demonstrated, and we sent a lot of patients south to our referral hospitals in Yellowknife or Edmonton.

Every month or two, letters began to arrive from Angelo, so I knew what was happening to him. Ron and I were very pleased to learn that his incarceration in Italy did not last very long. We knew that Barbara had left Canada to join him in Italy, and we very much hoped that they would find a place somewhere to settle down and continue with their life together. We secretly hoped that they might show up in Ottawa for our wedding in December.

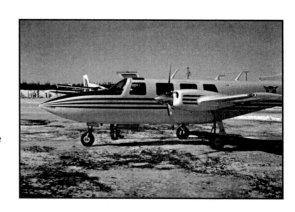

Ron's favourite plane for med-evacs, the Aerostar.

Arctic House Call: July 1976

The phone rang in my hospital office one day as I was doing paperwork.

"Dr. Lacroix?" the voice said, "We have a sick native woman at a fishing camp and we would like you to come to see her."

An arctic house call?

"Why not bring her to hospital?" I said.

"She refuses to come," he answered, "We can fly you here in our company helicopter; her husband has worked for us for many years. It's not very far."

I was speaking to the representative of a well-known oil exploration company, and realized that the patient's husband must be a highly regarded employee.

"Okay," I said.

"A company worker will pick you up at the hospital and take you to the base."

I grabbed my first aid bag and was met at the front door by the company employee. The helicopter was waiting at the airport and I was excited because I had never been in a helicopter before.

"This is the pilot, Beverly," said my host as he introduced me to a young man.

Beverly. Most unusual; Beverly was a woman's name. Must be English, I thought.

"Where's the Doctor?" he asked, "I was told there was a woman and a doctor coming?"

"There's just me, _I am_ the doctor," I answered, smiling at our mutual assumptions.

The pilot, Bev, the patient's husband, Frank, and I all climbed aboard the small bubble-shaped glass helicopter, floor transparent under our feet.

The engine roared, the blades beat the air above our heads and slowly the earth receded from underneath us. Trees around us shrank and we hovered just above their tops, moving horizontally. It was a most strange and wondrous sensation. We travelled this way for perhaps five minutes until Frank guided us to his fishing camp. Slowly, we set down in a small clearing between thin lodgepole pine trees.

Several tents with wooden walls and canvas roofs were set up along an arm of the Mackenzie River delta. Two large canoes rested on the marshy shores and a fire was smoking to dry fillets of fish on a wooden rack. Everything smelled of smoke.

Frank took me to see his wife, Daisy, a middle aged woman lying quietly on a cot in the tent. She seemed in a bit of pain, which for the stoic native people meant that she was in much distress. I examined her and concluded that she was having an attack of biliary colic or inflamed gallbladder. She would need surgery and we had no waiting lists.

"We must bring her back with us to the hospital," I said.

At this point Daisy agreed.

We crammed ourselves into the helicopter and flew straight up above the trees back to the airport. Then we took the patient to the hospital where our new surgeon, John, did a fine job of removing her gallbladder.

Daisy recovered very well and returned to her fishing camp home on the riverbank.

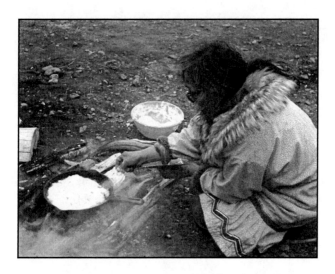

Making bannock at Arctic Summer Games.

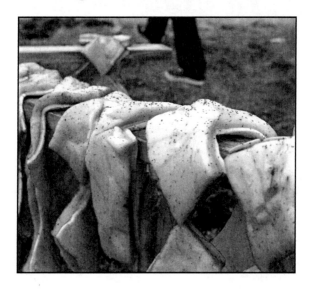

Muktuk (whale fat and skin), covered with flies, drying in the sun.

Bear Chase: September 1976

Fall came as it always does; the tundra turned bright red and gold amongst the spindly evergreens. Low fruit-covered bushes and a few bears could be seen in the wilderness surrounding the airport.

One day, as he returned from a flight, Ron asked me to meet him at the airport. I entered the small airport terminal building and asked Judy at the lunch counter whether she had seen Ron.

"He's at the hangar," she said, pointing to a large low building at the other end of the airport grounds about a block away.

"Thank you," I answered, "I'll walk over."

There were half a dozen people waiting inside the airport building, but the outside was completely deserted. I walked for a couple of minutes when some movement caught my eye. A black bear was casually walking in my direction about a block away, near the hangar. It was just a juvenile black bear, perhaps 3 feet high, but it was a bear, and he was coming in my direction.

I stopped and decided that I did not really want to cross his path so I turned around and started walking fairly quickly back to the airport building. I looked back and saw the bear was running in my direction.

This will not do, I thought to myself, and broke into a fine jog. Looking back one last time, I found the bear still heading my way. I stopped at the door to regain my composure, not wanting to scare anyone inside.

"There's a bear outside!" I said to Judy, trying not to sound too panicky.

"We know," she said, "He's around here all the time and he's harmless."

Shortly after, Ron showed up, laughing.

"We shooed the bear around towards the building," he said, "just to bug Judy, but we saw you running back to the terminal building and it was pretty funny. I guess our plan didn't work as well as we had hoped."

We all had a good laugh and the young bear happily returned to the woods.

Fall Snow: 1976

It had snowed all night, a real blizzard with sky and ground blending together, a white on white canvas. Ron had warmed up his car and left for the airport since he was on call that weekend; he would see if the weather had improved enough to allow a flight.

This was Saturday and I was not on call. My neighbor, Nancy, a public health nurse, asked me to walk with her to the store ten minutes away. I agreed since it would be good exercise. As usual I wore my fur parka, my wind pants, my fur mitts and big boots.

As Nancy and I walked past the igloo-shaped church over the snow covered sidewalk, a native man was waving at us from across the street.

"Hey, VD nurse," he yelled for all to hear.

VD was the acronym for venereal diseases, as sexually transmitted infections were known at the time.

"Hey, VD nurse, I'm ok now," he said loudly, not ashamed and likely not very sober in front of the half dozen people walking about.

"That's fine," Nancy waved back, laughing. VD was very common in town and the public health nurses were doing their best to track down and treat all cases.

We continued to the Hudson's Bay store and then to the post office where I picked up another of Angelo's letters. I walked back to my house eager to learn about the next events of our friend's life.

Ron and I had received the letter from Angelo announcing that he had split from Barbara. This was most unfortunate but somehow understandable. They made a lovely couple but she could not tolerate the uncertainty and exotic traveling of his lifestyle in countries that were very foreign to her. She wanted a home and a stable life. I could see that in her last letter. She was in Toronto, no doubt trying to heal a broken heart. She had come to the arctic looking for adventure and had perhaps found a stormy romance that was more complicated than she would have ever wished.

New Chief of Staff: Winter 1976-77

By the middle of the winter, I had become the senior doctor and Chief of Medical Staff; Maurice and Betty had moved to Nova Scotia. Several new young doctors had joined our team as our old friends finished their contracts and moved south to start new lives. Somehow the new recruits did not strike the same chord in our hearts as our previous friends, probably because Ron and I were planning our future elsewhere.

It seemed strange to me that I was no longer the greenhorn doctor. I had become the seasoned four-year veteran of our small arctic hospital. Being a senior doctor was not as much fun for me as being new; I always enjoyed my fresh new experiences, they remained clear in my mind, whereas the repeated ones all blend together.

Most of the medical staff had changed, so that by the time winter arrived in 1976, just a few months after Angelo's departure, nobody at the hospital talked about him anymore. As far as the hospital was concerned, Angelo DiStefano had sailed into history.

When total darkness returned to the land, one more time, in December, Ron and I flew to Ottawa for several weeks to prepare for our wedding.

We were married at Christmas with a simple ceremony and about 40 friends and relatives in attendance. While we had invited all our Inuvik friends, only Tom, Ron's pilot friend, and his wife Andrea, managed to make the trip. Bill sent me a lovely letter from his home in Alberta saying that he was very happy in his own marriage and wished us the same.

It somehow seemed appropriate for me to get married wearing a simple long pale pink gown, not white, as I had seen enough white in the arctic. I wore my fur parka and carried white and pink roses. I was delighted to see old friends from my Fort George days and Monique and Denis from my medical school days. I remembered Monique's prediction that she "saw me with a young man of German descent"; Ron's grandparents had, indeed, immigrated to Canada from German-speaking Austria.

I greatly enjoyed my large family during this particular Christmas; the many decorations, the Church midnight mass, the turkey, the tourtières, presents, noise and laughter.

Lianne Lacroix

By January 1977, Ron and I returned to Inuvik, back for one last tour of the cold and dark arctic. We were planning to move closer to Ron's family near Vancouver by the coming fall; the novelty of experiencing total darkness was completely gone and we longed for leafy trees and flowers once again.

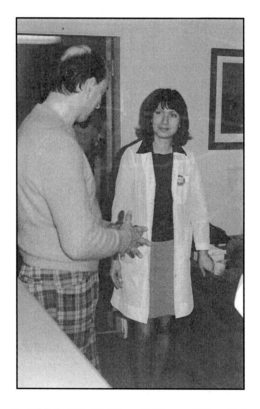

**As Chief of Staff at Inuvik General Hospital,
with Marc Lalonde, then Federal Minister of Health.**

Siamese Cat: Sachs Harbour, February 1977

Our last arctic winter lasted many months, as cold and dark as always. Then, slowly, a few daylight hours crept above the horizon, bringing the promise of a far away spring.

At this late date in our northern experience, I visited the village of Sachs Harbour, our northernmost outreach village. To get there, we had to fly over the Arctic Ocean for 325 miles, to the settlement on southern coast of Banks Island. The doctor who usually visited was away for some reason. The town had a nursing station building but was too small to have a permanent nurse.

The nurse that always accompanied the Sachs doctor would go with me. Eileen was a blue eyed, dark haired woman of Irish decent, in her early forties. She was competent and polite, but not friendly.

Perhaps she had a difficult childhood, I thought. She had been hurt and had closed her heart to the world for fear of pain; I enjoyed reading self-help psychology books and tried to understand people.

As we sat in the plane waiting to leave, an Inuit lady ran up and placed at our feet a cage containing a Siamese cat. Security was of little concern at the time.

The lady said, "Take this cat to Bella C., it belongs to her," and off she went with no further explanation. The cat was none too happy and let us know with his loud meows. I realized I had never seen a cat in the arctic. The poor scared feline entertained us with loud ear piercing calls drowning out the dull hum of the plane engines for the whole two hour flight. Fortunately Bella showed up to collect her cat as soon as we landed in Sachs. We never did find out the rest of that strange story.

Eileen and I were then driven to the nursing station. We slept in sleeping bags and kept the fire going in the small stove and tended to the half dozen patients that showed up the next morning. We had seen our last patient by early afternoon, and happily noted that it was still light outside. Some local villagers asked us if we wanted to ride as passengers on their skidoos to see the caribou. Large herds of Arctic Caribou had appeared near town that year; people were able to get quite close to them, but did not shoot unless it was necessary for food.

I grabbed my heavy 35 mm camera and hung it around my neck over my fur parka as we set off. After only ten minutes, we came upon a small group of three or four caribou walking around. They were large pale brown deer-of-the-north. We stared in amazement and they just stared back at us. They were not afraid.

I quickly took one photo and, as I manually advanced the film, I heard a snap and knew right away that the film had broken. Of course, film becomes very brittle at 40° below zero, so I never did capture pictures of those caribou. No matter, for we gazed for a few minutes at the magnificent beasts, then quickly returned to our warm shelters.

The next day, Eileen and I returned to Inuvik. I never did find out anything more about her; she left the north shortly thereafter and I suspect she did not find what she was looking for. The north brings many people searching for many things, whether freedom, adventure or love. Some are running away from situations down south or have found that they are just too different to fit in with regular society. Many were just passing through; restless hearts without a home, looking for the comfort they never knew in their own childhoods. For them, the arctic held no magic; the bleak winds chilled their fragile hearts, so they would move on and head back south.

Glimmer of Hope: June1977

Winter eventually melted into spring, and summer soon arrived, bringing the usual dust and mosquitoes. Many hospital staff left for holidays and the *summer people* arrived once more. Students came to study arctic lands and search for natural resources. That summer we noticed geologists looking for diamonds and government officials continued talking about building a gas pipeline across the barren lands.

Every month I continued to visit Aklavik, spending two or three days treating patients at the nursing station. By now Liz had moved south to work in public health and wrote to me that she was happy with her new boyfriend. Iris had left her nursing job and assimilated into the local community by marrying her Inuit boyfriend.

The nursing station welcomed a nurse named Julie who was very friendly. She even called me by my first name, which I found a bit unnerving as by now I was very used to the name "doctor".

I saw the same local people that I had seen many times over the past four years, I witnessed their daily struggles fighting poverty, violence, depression and alcoholism. As the years passed, nothing much seemed to change for them.

On this visit, as the afternoon clinic was coming to an end, the phone rang. Julie answered, listened for a moment, and relayed the information to me. "Lianne, we have an 18 year old woman called Clara coming right over and she's bleeding."

I knew Clara was three months pregnant. I did not need to ask what kind of bleeding she was experiencing. "She's most likely having a miscarriage," I answered.

Sure enough, after I examined Clara, I said to Julie, "We'll have to call for a plane to take her to the hospital. She can't wait until tomorrow for the sched."

This was the scheduled plane that I normally took when returning to Inuvik. Julie called the hospital to arrange a med-evac.

By now it was early evening on a quiet summer day; the sun was slowly sinking into a light pink sky.

We prepared Clara for the trip by starting an IV and placing her on a stretcher, since she was in danger of suffering a major hemorrhage. She would likely need a D&C (dilation and curettage) which would be performed by our surgeon.

Within an hour we heard a plane circling over town, preparing to land on the runway, just across the road from the Aklavik nursing station.

With the stretcher on the floor of our station wagon we quickly made our way to the airstrip.

The Cessna 185 landed very expertly and slowly came to a stop just in front of us. The plane door opened and the pilot jumped out. It was a young woman! I stared in surprise. I had never seen a female pilot in the arctic! Suppressing my delight, I introduced myself and she answered, "My name is Diane and I'm your pilot today."

We carefully loaded Clara's stretcher into the plane, making sure that it was tied down with seatbelts. Then I climbed aboard beside Diane. She turned the plane and flew back towards Inuvik, over the multitude of meandering channels in the Mackenzie River delta.

During the twenty minute trip back to town, I tried hard not to ask too many questions as I did not want to distract her from her work. I learned that she came from Fort Smith and was working in town for the summer to gain experience and accumulate flying hours. She appeared to be around twenty-five years old and her dark brown eyes suggested a possible Metis ancestry, I thought, but I had no time to ask.

Here we were, three young women alone in a plane - a pilot, a doctor and a patient, and I wondered if it was perhaps the first time that the arctic had witnessed a med-evac staffed by all female professionals. I rather enjoyed every moment of that short flight.

Soon we were landing and loading Clara into the hospital station wagon. I waved to Diane as we drove off down the gravel road, still bordered by spindly evergreens. I felt that something very different had happened that day and I knew in that moment that I had caught a glimpse of the future when planes would be piloted not only by local men but also by local aboriginal women. Indeed I felt certain that some of the children that I had delivered in the arctic would grow up to be pilots and doctors and whoever else was needed to improve the lives of the people of this land.

Baby Angel: July 1977

Summer was very hot with no wind at all. The sun traveled continually around the sky with no reprieve of darkness. The thermometer climbed over 80° Fahrenheit. It seemed ironic to be caught in a heat wave so far north of the Arctic Circle, even if it was the height of summer.

It was close to midnight and I was just getting ready for bed when the phone rang. It was Chipo. "Elisa just showed up in strong labour," she said, calm as always. "She's 8cm dilated."

"Be right over," I answered, ready as always.

I jumped into my jeans and cotton top and jogged the two blocks to the hospital.

Elisa was a young native woman of mixed European-Inuit ancestry who was caught in the world of drugs and alcohol. She had come to the hospital for only one pre-natal visit and would not accept all the help that was offered to her.

I reached the quiet hospital, knowing that Chipo was the only nurse on night duty in the obstetric ward. As I turned the last corner I could hear screaming and swearing, "Make this f---ing pain stop! Make this f---ing pain stop!"

At the door of the birthing room, I quickly evaluated the situation. Elisa was totally out of control, yelling and thrashing with her arms flailing in the air. Chipo was stuck between Elisa's legs, pushing them apart while she tried to hold the baby's small blue head which was strangling as she was being born.

I felt concern for both the poor baby and overwrought Elisa. With no hesitation, as if by reflex, I walked over and grabbed Elisa tightly and held her in my arms as she struggled and then quickly relaxed. Chipo managed to finish delivering the small baby.

"I'm sorry you guys," Elisa kept repeating over and over as she regained some of her senses.

"You have a beautiful girl," said Chipo as we resuscitated the small child in the bassinet. She cried within one minute and seemed ready to survive.

We cleaned up and took the baby to the nursery while Elisa rested in a room. Chipo and I reviewed the scene and we both felt that we had done our best under difficult circumstances.

The next day Elisa wanted to leave the hospital. "I don't want the baby," she said, "you keep it."

We asked James, the quiet spoken social worker, to come and talk with her. She was adamant that she wanted to leave and signed herself out of the hospital against medical advice.

James took over legal guardianship of the tiny delicate baby girl that the nurses in the nursery named Angel. She cried little and fed poorly and the nurses soon noticed that she turned blue whenever she cried.

All of the doctors listened to her heart and lungs during our weekly rounds. She must have congenital heart disease, we concluded. This meant that her heart had not formed normally before she was born.

A couple of weeks later when Angel was judged strong enough to survive the trip, we sent her to Edmonton to see some specialists.

We heard nothing for a few more weeks. Our only means of communication were letters and telephone calls. The hospital did not have a fax machine as they were not yet in common use in the mid-1970's.

Then one day a nurse returning from holidays brought two month old Angel back to us. She was beautiful and alert but remained very small.

Attached to her blankets by a large safety pin we found a long typed letter from the specialists, who explained that she had been born with three chambers in her heart instead of the normal four. She had only one ventricle and there was nothing that they could do. Heart transplants for infants were not available at the time. She was not expected to live much longer.

James said, "I will try to reach Elisa to let her know, in case she wants to come to see her." Elisa never showed up.

The nurses in the pediatric ward looked after Angel and, when not too busy, could be seen rocking the baby in an old rocking chair.

Even our young new doctor, Jacques, a curly haired marathon runner who always wore unlaced running shoes, would rock Angel when times were quiet.

A few weeks passed. Then one morning Jacques reported to us, with tears in his eyes, that little Angel had flown to heaven. She had died during the night and we all grieved for a moment for the tiny life that had graced our days just like the short arctic summer that was fast disappearing into the fall.

Liquor Store Plebiscite: Summer 1977

Thursday morning rounds, followed by a lunch meeting in the boardroom to discuss medical problems, were an IGH tradition. Now the Chief of Staff, I looked around the long boardroom table at the new doctors sitting where Bill, Ronald and Angelo had sat just a year or two before.

"Our biggest medical problem is alcoholism," I said, and we all knew it very well. "I wish there was something that we could do to help."

"We must do something," said Colin, one of the new recruits. "How about picketing the liquor store?"

"No, that would not help, and we are to busy looking after the patients affected by this illness," answered John, our young surgeon.

"We need to close the liquor store," said Jacques, who had cradled baby Angel.

"I agree totally," I answered. "I read that Frobisher Bay (an eastern arctic town) did that last year and it has helped."

"Then we need a detox centre," added Colin, "and counselors too."

We certainly all agreed, but what could we do?

The room was silent for a few seconds as we contemplated the massive problem. I remembered the numerous patients whose lives had been shattered by alcohol; the young man in the eastern arctic who died in front of my eyes, the young woman burned in her cabin, baby Angel, and so many others…so much suffering…we could think of no other solutions.

"What can we do? We are only doctors," said John.

"We could start by writing a letter to "The Drum" (our local newspaper) expressing our concern," I said finally.

They all agreed and, since it was my idea, I volunteered to write it.

"Close Inuvik Liquor Store"

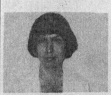

Dr. L. Lacroix, Inuvik General Hospital.

Editor's Note: L. Lacroix, M.D. has served delta residents for many years. Below, Dr. Lacroix writes of "people whose lives and health are being destroyed by drinking." Inside, beginning on page 2, The DRUM carries a summary of a study of the changes observed in the lifestyle of Frobisher Bay residents after the closing of their liquor store on April 30, 1976.

The Editor "The DRUM"

Having worked here for almost four years as a medical doctor, I have not failed to notice the north's greatest medical problem — alcoholism.

Every day in the hospital we see so many people whose lives and health are being destroyed by drinking. Their brain is being permanently damaged by alcohol so that they can no longer think properly. Their nerves are overexcited. Whenever they stop drinking, they shake so much that they must have another drink. They fall down and hurt themselves or freeze to death in the winter. They get into fights, cut their heads and faces, bleed all over and run to the hospital for stitches. Their houses burn down through carelessness. Sometimes they knife or shoot each other to

death. The N.W.T. has the highest murder rate in Canada. I have seen quite a few of these useless deaths in the last four years.

People who drink too much cannot find or hold jobs, their families have no food or clothes. Their neglected children get sick and must be admitted to hospital when all they need is a good home. Their families break up. With such parents the children grow up to become drunks too.

It is quite a sad picture. The future looks pretty grim for the people of this town and surrounding settlements. With so much liquor around how can anyone say no to drinking when all his friends drink too.

If only there were some way of stopping the flow of alcohol to this part of the country, it would help. This has been done in other parts Continued from page 2

My letter was published in "The Drum'" on Wednesday July 20, 1977 as follows:

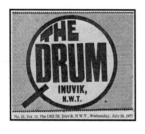

"Close Inuvik Liquor Store"

Having worked here for almost four years as a medical doctor, I have not failed to notice the north's greatest medical problem- alcoholism.

Every day in the hospital we see so many people whose lives and health are being destroyed by drinking. Their brain is being permanently damaged by alcohol so that they can no longer think properly. Their nerves are overexcited. Whenever they stop drinking they shake so much that they must have another drink. They fall down and hurt themselves or freeze to death in winter. They get into fights, cut their heads and faces, bleed all over and run to the hospital to get stitches. Their houses burn down through carelessness. Sometimes they knife or shoot each other to death. The N.W.T. has the highest murder rate in Canada. I have seen quite a few of these useless deaths in the last four years.

People who drink too much cannot hold or find jobs; their families have no food or clothes. Their neglected children get sick and must be admitted to the hospital when all they need is a good home. Their families break up. With such parents the children grow up to become drunks too.

It is quite a sad picture. The future looks pretty grim for the people of this town and surrounding settlements. With so much liquor around how can anyone say no to drinking when all their friends drink too.

If only there was some way of stopping the flow of alcohol to this part of the country, it would help. This has been done in other parts of the north. The people of Frobisher Bay held a plebiscite in the summer of 1976 and the majority agreed to close down the liquor store. Already the health of that town has improved.

We could do the same in this town. We could close down the liquor store. Surely no one wants to watch people suffering and killing themselves from drinking. It is such a terrible waste. When in the bush or working in the oil rigs people don't drink-they can do without it. When they come to town the bars could be open for those who enjoy listening to music with friends and a drink or two. But no liquor would be available at home so that weeks-long drinking sprees would no longer be possible. If there were no liquor store in this town the alcoholism would surely decrease.

I ask everybody to think about this. If the people of this town got together in a plebiscite and closed down the liquor store, the plague of alcoholism would be slowed down. Then someday the people of the north would no longer be slaves to their drinking but free to live their own lives in good heath and happiness.

L. Lacroix
Chief of Staff, Inuvik General Hospital,
Inuvik N.W.T.

A couple of weeks later Corrine said, "Dr. Lacroix, there is a call for you from James."

James was the social worker who had been the legal guardian of baby Angel. I answered the phone.

"Dr. Lacroix, I am calling about your letter in the newspaper. I would like to invite you to come and talk about this. Don't tell anyone. This is secret," he said.

He then gave me a time and a place, which turned out to be the government office. I showed up at the designated time a few days later and knocked on the office door. James let me into a non-descript beige office and showed me to a room where four other people were sitting around a table.

I recognized Susie, a local native social worker who was well respected, but none of the other people. James introduced me to a teacher, a public health nurse and a male native town representative.

"We are the 'Committee of the Concerned'," he said.

"Why the secrecy?" I asked.

"Because most of us work for the government and when we were hired we signed a paper saying that we would not get involved in local affairs, or we might get fired."

This clause must have been drafted many decades ago to try to minimize the influence of Europeans on the local native people, I thought. And now it was too late; the damage was done with the introduction of alcohol, and it was clear that we must now do all we can to help. A threat to my job did not seem much of a concern to me.

"Count me in," I told them.

We agreed that closing the liquor store was a good idea and we started to plan the details of the plebiscite which would be required in order to close the liquor store.

We met a few more times and drew up a petition to be circulated around town. Within a few weeks we had collected 765 names and sent them to Commissioner Stuart Hodgson, requesting a plebiscite. Many articles and letters for and against appeared in "The Drum" during this time. The members of the Legion were against the idea while medical and educational personnel were all very much in favour.

Finally, just as Ron and I were preparing to leave in the fall of 1977, everything came together and a plebiscite was held in Inuvik asking the citizens if they wanted to close the liquor store. The majority voted against the idea; the people of Inuvik had spoken.

We had lost. The 'Committee of the Concerned' was disappointed but not surprised; we had started the dialogue, and brought the subject out in the open. I like to think that we lit a candle that flickered for one brief moment, shedding light on the darkness of alcoholic despair, and that someday it would re-ignite and lead a desperate people back to good health and self respect.

My Last Arctic Patient: October 1977

The time had come for Ron and I to leave and start a new chapter in our lives. We looked forward to being closer to our families and starting a family of our own. The adventure was over, and we could feel it; we did not belong in the north anymore.

I was expecting to leave quietly, reflecting on my four year adventure as we traveled south, but of course such was not to be the case.

By then, Ron, who was a professional pilot, had bought a small single engine Piper Comanche, for personal use. This plane was much too advanced for me to fly, so I was content to focus on map reading.

It was October, 1977, and the weather was rainy with strong winds, and it was getting colder. There was not a lot of snow on the ground yet, but winter was fast approaching. After carefully observing the weather, we took off and flew south about 500 miles, landing at

Norman Wells to refuel.

The bad weather was closing in. "The weather doesn't look good," said Ron, "I think we'll stay here for a while. We'll have to wait for the system to pass through."

"Okay," I said. We decided to wait at the small airport, and if the weather did not improve, we would go to the local hotel.

The Norman Wells airport waiting room was not very large. We were the only ones waiting and we could see and hear all that was going on. There was a large Armed Forces Hercules rescue plane parked at one end of the tarmac. We knew that two days before, a small plane had gone missing on its way from Inuvik to Yellowknife. The pilot was a young RCMP officer who had recently learned to fly. He had been taking his girlfriend to Yellowknife to attend the RCMP ball. The weather deteriorated as he left, bringing snow showers and winds. The young couple never reached their destination.

Two army personnel strode through the waiting room towards the manager's office at one end. "They've found the plane!" one man exclaimed. "There's one survivor and the helicopter is bringing him out. Can you call the nursing station and ask the nurse to accompany the patient to Yellowknife?" he said.

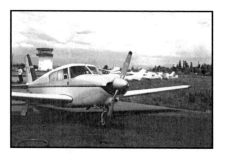

**Piper Commanche,
our personal plane.**

I knew that the nurse at Norman Wells would not be too keen to leave her town unattended. I could overhear the conversation.

"This must be my cue," I said to Ron. I could not ignore the situation, although I admit I hesitated for a moment. I walked over to them.

"Hi," I said, "I'm a local doctor passing through and could accompany your patient to Yellowknife."

"Great," they exclaimed.

"This is my husband, Ron," I said. "He's a pilot too and is coming with us."

"Sure," they said.

Within an hour the helicopter had landed with the patient. I grabbed my first aid bag from our plane and walked to the large Hercules plane.

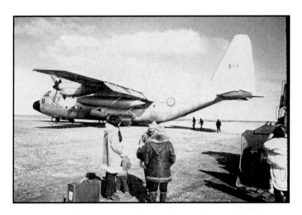

Canadian Armed Forces Hercules plane.

Inside, it looked like a hangar, or maybe a garage or a large bus with all the seats removed. It was unheated and unfinished. The patient was lying quietly on a stretcher along one wall, with a search and rescue medic by his side. I did a quick assessment. The patient seemed conscious, quiet and calm. He answered simple questions with yes or no. I immediately noticed that one pupil was dilated, which meant it was enlarged and not moving. He was dressed in heavy outdoor clothing, winter parka and heavy pants, and no blood was visible. I certainly would not remove any clothes; the inside of the large plane was just above freezing and I felt 'just comfortable' in my fur parka. I palpated his head and felt some lumpy areas the size of my fist. He obviously had a severe head injury; the lumpy areas were surely a skull fracture. I felt his arms and legs. They were all uneven and irregular. I concluded that he had two broken legs near the ankles and had two broken arms.

The medic told me that they found the plane crashed upside down with the wounded man hanging by his seatbelt. His girlfriend was dead beside him. He had been waiting 48 hours for rescue, and it was an absolute miracle that he was still alive. Likely his heavy clothes and heavy build helped to preserve his body heat. He was suffering from exposure and his body temperature was lower than normal. He was conscious, but in shock; his body had almost shut down, which is why he seemed so calm and detached; most of his brain was not working.

My diagnosis was head injury, skull fracture, two broken legs, two broken arms, dehydration and shock, with likely internal injuries. "What could I possibly do to help him?" I asked myself.

Then I asked the medic, "Do you have any IV solution?"

"Yes," he answered, "We have ringers." (standard salt water and sugar solution used in Emergencies)

"I'll put in an IV," I said. I looked in my first aid bag and found my 16-gauge medicuts, a plastic tube connected to a 16-gauge needle. I lifted his sleeves and searched for a vein. His hands and arms were cold. No veins at all. I tried several times with my needle, no luck. The patient did not flinch, as if he felt nothing.

A gentle hand on my shoulder. Ron's voice, "The pilots are ready to go if you are."

"Yes, tell them to go," I answered. "Getting this man to the hospital as fast as we can is the best thing we can do."

Yellowknife was two hours away and the weather was poor. The big Hercules plane started to move down the taxiway groaning and shaking. I was determined to get an IV going. I tried again and again. Everything shook. The wounded man just lay there quietly, looking straight ahead, oblivious to everything. Finally in the *cubital fossa*, the crook of the elbow, I hit a vein and some dark blood came out, properly nestling my plastic needle.

I said to the medic, "Do we have anything to warm up the IV solution?"

It was room temperature, not far above zero, and I was trying to warm it up with my bare hands. The medic came back with a warm towel and we wrapped the solution up in it.

Just then the big plane lumbered down the runway and slowly took off, gaining altitude in the cloudy, gray, bumpy sky.

I sat beside the patient, hoping that he would survive until we reached the hospital. He said nothing, but would still answer simple questions appropriately. I wondered if he knew what had happened to him. He could not answer that. Did he know that his girlfriend was dead? I could not ask.

We finally landed and made our way to the Yellowknife Hospital where I transferred his care to the doctor on call. X-rays confirmed the various severe fractures. The next day, the patient was evacuated by plane to Edmonton to begin his long recovery. I never did hear what happened to him and would suspect that he suffers from serious residual effects to this day.

That night, Ron and I found a local hotel where we slept, exhausted, as the bad weather system rolled by.

The skies were clear the next morning and Search and Rescue arranged for us to catch a flight back to Norman Wells. We returned to our own small plane and our own journey south.

Dark grey clouds dissipated as the miles rolled away under our plane. Evergreen forests gave way to small fields and a few buildings started to appear along the rivers. Ron and I felt very quiet and said little.

We were reflecting on all our experiences working in the north and the friends that had come and gone. We marveled at how we had found each other. We had the feeling that our time in the north was really over now and that a new life was waiting for us somewhere else.

Far beneath us, the dull brown land turned to lush green fields and columns of light from the bright sun guided us towards the next chapter of our lives. We looked back one more time. The arctic was vanishing behind great clouds of snow just as those memories would slowly fade like a dream.

Roses and Babies: Summer 1979

Two years had passed since I had spent those four memorable years in the arctic.

Ron and I were very busy in our new life near Vancouver where we lived on an acre of land filled with magnificent trees including a peach tree and several large climbing pink roses that bloomed in early summer. It was my favourite time of the year; roses were blooming everywhere and their sweet perfume filled the air. Indeed we had planted a rose garden of some thirty bushes and I even belonged to the local rose society. Every day I enjoyed their fragile beauty, symbolic of the quick passage of time.

Ron was flying twenty-passenger Twin Otters on floats for Air West, a company that eventually became Air BC and was later absorbed by Air Canada. He travelled every day to the airport and was working hard, enjoying the friendship of his flying colleagues.

I worked half time at a nearby medical clinic and delivered many babies at the local community hospital at all hours of the day and night. Ron and I were blessed by the birth of our beautiful blue-eyed daughter. She learned to crawl on the lush green lawn of our pleasant home. Her little toddler feet carried her over a small wooden bridge to the garden where she walked with me among the roses.

We seldom thought about the arctic anymore. Every Christmas I looked through my address book and mailed cards to our old friends. It was this way that Angelo's last two letters came to me. Afterwards my cards went unanswered...

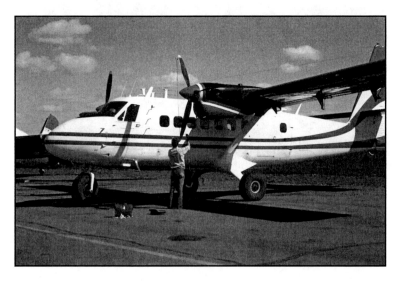

DeHavilland Twin Otter.

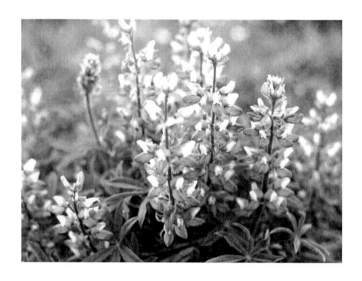

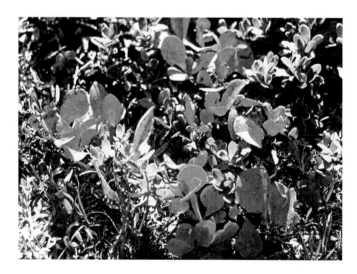

Eight

The Key To the Whole Story: 1984

The elevator door I was patiently waiting for at Kelowna General Hospital slowly opened and out stepped a distinguished grey-haired man. It was 1984 and I was now living and working in the Okanagan Valley.

"Why Dr. Lacroix," he exclaimed, "I have not seen you since you left the arctic."

I recognized him right away. He was Mr. Harkness, the second in command at the Northern Health Ministry. He had been stationed in Edmonton and looked after hiring doctors for Inuvik General Hospital. He had visited us in Inuvik several times.

"Quite a story about that surgeon who was arrested as an impostor," he said.

"Yes, he was my friend," I answered.

"It was his wife, you know, she reported him to the authorities! Not happy about their divorce most likely," he said.

I was speechless for a moment. It all made sense now. Angelo's wife, Stella, had come to visit him in the arctic only a few months before he was arrested. But why had she come? He had told us that they were separated and that he was free. Perhaps Stella viewed their marriage differently and hoped they would get back together. She had obviously discovered that Angelo was involved in a new relationship and it probably did not help that the new woman was a very beautiful, younger blonde.

It seems that Stella could not accept that her marriage was over and felt terribly hurt; she wanted revenge. Perhaps she had hoped that Angelo would eventually return to her and their teenaged daughter after his long sojourns for training overseas. But after her visit to Canada, she reported her husband to the Italian authorities who then contacted Canadian authorities to have him extradited back to Italy. Did she hope that he would linger in prison, that she could ruin his life?

Somehow, the small Italian boy who had survived the war years in his ravaged country would never be defeated by hate. He had survived poverty and hunger and spent a lifetime fighting for what he felt was right.

Angelo would not spend long in prison. At just the right time for him, Italy elected a Communist government and Angelo had regained his freedom. He found work in a tropical country far from the arctic snows. He soon found love with Eliana and remarried. She gave him a fine son and as he mentioned to me in his last letter, he was "happy in a land that is always sunny."

As the elevator door closed, Mr. Harkness said goodbye and walked away, leaving me with memories of the north flooding into my mind. It all made sense to me now.

Where are they now?

What happened to the people that we met in the arctic so long ago?

Ronald Calderisi became a very well respected general surgeon in Vancouver. He was revered by his patients for his compassion and skill. He returned to work in the arctic at the end of his career and did volunteer work in Africa and the Arab States. Sadly he passed away suddenly from heart disease in 2005 at the age of 56.

Bill and Shirley still live in the mountains of Alberta where they run a bed and breakfast. Bill practices medicine and anaesthetic at his local hospital. They have two adult children.

Barbara married two years after leaving Inuvik and lives with her family in the Toronto area.

Chipo married an armed forces officer, adopted an Inuit baby and moved to Ottawa where she opened a beauty spa.

We have lost track of all the other people that we once knew. Life is like the wind on a warm autumn day; it blows together piles of leaves that share the experience of a moment in time and space, and then another gust of wind blows the leaves apart, spreading them in all directions, never to touch again...

When I started writing this book a few years ago, I began searching for Angelo. I have searched the internet and found nothing. I have written to the three addresses that he had given me in Italy and Venezuela. There was no answer. He had told me that his aunt in his home town of Serracapriola, Italy, would know where he was living. I sent a letter there. It came back saying that she is deceased. I was in touch with the Italian Medical Association and they had not heard of him.

He would now be over 70 years old and likely retired, although I cannot imagine that Angelo would stop working unless his health forced him to slow down. I like to think that he is living in a sunny Italian villa surrounded by his children and grandchildren. Perhaps he is reflecting on his life, where he fought for the poor against injustice and saved many lives as a surgeon. I hope that Angelo has found true love and contentment in the sunset years of his life.

21 - XI - 76

Dear Lianne,

je bien reçu votre invitation pour le mariage - je veu deux - une o Sorrecap avola et autre chez mon frere - je vous remercie de Toute mon cœur, mais pour moi c'est impossible pouvoir venir o votre mariage pour différent raison - le premiere c'est que le 2 de Decembre je dois disouter la Thesis - et aussitôt après probablement je part pour compte du Gouvernement Italienne au service du Ministere avec l'exterieur pour l'aide aux pays du 3em monde - c'est possible que on m'envoye en Afrique au

Augurri,
Loa e gle

Nine: Attachments

The letters and postcards of Angelo DiStefano are presented in chronological order as I received them while living in Inuvik and near Vancouver. They explain what happened to him after he left the arctic. Some were written in French and I have translated them. My comments are inserted in italics. I am publishing these very private and personal letters so that the truth is known about the surgeon unjustly called impostor in order to preserve the memory of his competent surgical work.

Item:	Sent from:	Dated:
Angelo: Letter 1	Rome	March 24, 1976
Angelo: Letter 2	Rome	March 27, 1976
Angelo: Letter 3	Rome	April 15, 1976
Postcard 1	Rome	May 14, 1976
Postcard 2	Milano	May 15, 1976
Postcard 3	Serracapriola	May 30, 1976
Angelo: Letter 4	New York	June 14, 1976
Angelo: Letter 5	New York	June 20, 1976
Barbara: Letter 1	Toronto	July 21, 1976
Barbara: Letter 2	Toronto	July 23, 1976
Angelo: Letter 6	Italy	October 31, 1976
Angelo: Letter 7	Rome	November 21, 1976
Angelo: Letter 8	Rome	January 30, 1977
Angelo: Letter 9	Rome	April 4, 1978
Postcard 4	Rome	Christmas, 1978
Angelo: Letter 10	Venezuela	March 3, 1981

Article: "Unmasking Bogus Doctors"		September, 1982
Letter to Editor from Lianne Lacroix		September, 1982
Letter from Bill Sara		October 5, 1982

Angelo's Letters
Number 1: from Rome

Dated March 24, 1976
Rome Political detainee cell 26

Dear Lianne and Ron:

This is my third letter to you but no answer (*we never received them*). I think you are very busy, well, I wish to thank you very much for all the efforts that you are doing for me.

Barbara, which thanks God I start receiving some news, she keeps me informed of what my friends are doing in my favour... very nice...I will never forget.

My dear Lianne, the life here is very hard for me in this prison. I am a political prisoner and I am allowed to have a radio and television if I own them. I am allowed to have almost everything like a watch and personal items.

But I am very depressed because even my daughter, she never came to see me, I am very alone. The only comfort comes from Barbara and you must know that she is all my life and I must be strong for her, because my life has no value in here.

As you know on March 3, I arrived at Fiumicino Airport in Rome with the Police. The police brought me to Questura Central office of Rome Police. They freed me from the charge of extradition and invited me to go home- but in my way to go – at the second floor- the Political Police stopped me and notified me of the real reason for my arrest! --"Conspiracy against the State" and Fall in sevbitious (*illegible*)---for this charge I was convicted in absence two years after leaving the country. But I have heard the prosecutor say that she wants to offer mercy---Few days ago the lawyer says that the Police wants to charge me too because they think that I was an agent of the CIA in Italy!!!

Lianne , believe me I AM INNOCENT. I am in this prison innocent, I am never doing these things. Few days ago I wrote the CBC and the Drum *(local Inuvik newspaper)* to say that they must stop insulting me and there are investigations looking into all.

Well, on May 18 the Appeal will come but not in public, nobody including the press will know what is happening to me, what these people are doing to me—this is incredible. Italy is today worst than in Fascist times. The prison all over is very full of innocent people waiting for years and years for a crazy trial.

Well, Lianne I hope that soon it will end for me because there is a rumour that very soon the Government will give a general amnesty for political prisoners. I hope that this is true.

Please give my regards to Ron and tell him to write me sometimes. It will be very pleasant if you write to me and give me some news about Inuvik where is my heart.

Please Lianne keep close to Barbara for me. She is everything. I will be grateful to you if you help her if she needed some help. Hi to all our hospital friends.

With love,

Angelo

Angelo's Letters
Number 2: from Rome

Dated March 27 1976 Rome Political Prisoner cell 26

My dear Lianne;

It is with great joy that I received your letter today. I am so glad. Today was a good day for me....two letters from Barbara and one from Anna (*another nurse friend from Inuvik*) plus your letter. Here the only contact that we have with outside life are letters, like a bit of sunshine in this dark prison cell with no sunlight.

I am very sad because I love Barbara and I am very far from her and afraid of losing her. Lianne if I ever lose her, for me, my life is over.

Here I am alone, never any visitors except for today when my brother came. He came to talk about politics so I showed him the door and told him to not come to see me again in this prison. My daughter never came to see me and she goes to school only 500 meters from this prison. This hurts my heart—after many sacrifices to look after her for her future. I am alone like a dog and I have never hurt anybody but was always helping people and doing some good. Enfin c'est la vie...(*Anyhow that is life*)

I hope with all my heart to come to your wedding (*planned for December 1976*) and I hope to be free by July. The Court refuses me bail because Stella (*his ex-wife*) wrote a letter to the president (*of the court*) saying that I would run away to Canada to be with my new wife Barbara. She warned them to be very careful in granting me any freedom as I would likely not attend a court date in the future.

194

Say hello to Ron and I hope to see him soon. Please ask the hospital to send me my vacation pay and last pay because I need this money to pay my bills.

Au revoir, see you soon, stay close to Barbara please,

Your Angelo

Angelo's Letters
Number 3: from Rome

Dated April 15 1976
Rome Political Prisoner cell 26

Dear Lianne:

Thanks very much for a beautiful letter received today. My moral (*mood*) is good because I regularly receive mail from my wife Barbie. She is so sweet. I say she is the angel of my life. I am very happy no matter if I am in jail, I do not care. It will end soon I hope. But it is so nice to be in love no matter if at present we are 10,000 miles apart. Thanks God! For the first time in my life I am happy here in this condition. I think about when I will be free and with Barbie. No one can appreciate their own home more than after this separation.

Well, here it is the same life-- closed into a cell (*illegible*) watching for news, letters... On May 18, I have my appeal trial and I hope all will be OK. I have another lawyer, the second one. He is a Professor in Law and cost me a lot of money but no matter.

Stella (*ex-wife*) continues to trouble me but I do not care. She is going around to the Judge to tell so many things wrong about me. She said that I was a CIA agent!!! She's crazy. Thanks God the Judge does not believe her and acquitted me of this charge. We will see what happens.

The Italian economic and political situation is disastrous. Everything is wrong in this country. Many people are arrested everyday for nothing. We have a chance to have a general election on June 13 . There is a chance of a general amnesty for political prisoners. We will see what happens.

On April 27 I will go to Court for my final divorce- no problem for that I hope.

I hope to be free very soon. Barbara and I will come to see you right after I am free even if I have to travel to Inuvik. See you soon. You and Ron are my best friends.

Love, Angelo

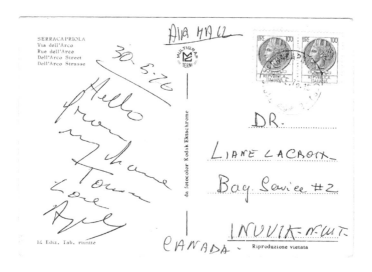

Postcard #3 from Angelo's hometown Serracapriola. May 30, 1976.

....

At the June 13, 1976 election a different party was elected in Italy and Angelo was given amnesty and regained his freedom. He sent me three postcards over the course of two weeks, from three separate locations:

1. From Rome dated May 14, 1976 saying:

"Rome, waiting for your honeymoon-with love...Angelo"

2. From Milano dated May 15, 1976 saying:

"Thanks for all with love ...Angelo"

3. From Serracapriola dated May 30, 1976 saying:

"Hello from my home town ...love Angelo"

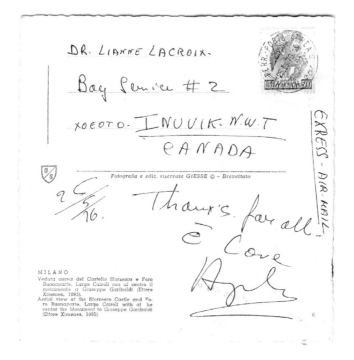

Angelo's Letters
Number 4: from New York

Dated June 14, 1976
New York USA

Dear Lianne:

I am in New York for more than a week with Barbara at my family's house in the mountain out of the city. We have good times.

This morning I went to Albany N. Y. at the Medical Board for endorsement of my Michigan licence in the N.Y. state. I will have probably a full licence by October. I will send the application in the next few days after receiving some documents from the Michigan Board *(medical)* in Lansing.

Well I think I will stay for good in New York state and open my own private practice with some group of other doctors. In October I will give my thesis in Rome. Finally the president of the Faculty Professor Einimo *(illegible)* gave me permission to present my dissertation of thesis.

Barbara and I not too good on Wednesday. She returned home. For that I must thank all - *(names of Canadian health officials)*. One day these people will tell me "I am sorry" for my troubles since I will write my thesis in October. I will sue a lot of people for slander. After I will see-no matter if I must work only to pay for lawyers.

Well I wish one time again to thank you for everything that you are doing for me. If you have a chance to see Father Lemire *(Inuvik priest)* please thank him for me.

Maybe I will go to Ottawa for a few days to talk with Dr

Larose *(health official)*.

Few days ago I went to Ottawa Consul to ask if I can get back to Canada.

I hope to see you soon. Regards and love to Ron

Your faithful, Angelo

Angelo's Letters
Number 5: from New York

Dated June 20, 1976
New York USA

Dear Lianne;

I am processing my endorsement of the Michigan licence to the New York State. For this purpose I need three supporting statements from three colleagues.

I will be grateful of you return to me the enclosed statement *(this was done)*.

I plan to stay in New York until October or March depending on the Canadian Government giving me permission to practice in Canada.

Hope that you have a nice holiday.

My best to Ron,

With Barb everything OK,

Hope hearing from you soon, with love Angelo

Letter from Barbara #1
Wednesday July 21 1976 Toronto, Ontario

Hello Lianne and Ron,

How are things in Inuvik? I suppose nothing much has changed. Thought I would just drop you a short line to let you know what's happening with Angelo and myself.

I think the last Angelo wrote to you, he was looking for a job in New York. Well he found a job and could get a temporary medical licence but could not get a working visa, not for some time anyways like six months or a year.

So he came up here and we went to Ottawa together and saw Dr. Laroche (*Health official*) about all this 'psychopath' matter[2]. Well Dr. Laroche was very nice and said that he and Dr Black really had no doubt that Angelo was a qualified Doctor but they were just going by what the University of Rome said.

So Angelo gave them the names of his professors and the Registrar of the Medical school (Rome) and told them to check it again. So they were going to get the government in Rome to look into it.

Dr. Laroche said at one point in this story it did look like Angelo was a 'psychopath' like the 'great impostor' but as more of the story came out, he found that there were explanations for things.

Then Peter Smith Director of Personnel (*Health and Welfare*) came and saw Angelo. He seemed very interested in rehiring Angelo. He said as far as they are concerned Angelo has a

---

[2] The word psychopath was used in reference to the "great impostor", a man called Fred Demara, who deceived many people with his masquerade as a doctor along with many other professions. Such a man has no conscience and does not care for the feeling of others which was certainly NOT the case with Angelo.

clear record with them and an excellent clinical record. As far as they are concerned now, all he needs is a licence from one of the provinces and his landed immigrant status which he has. As for the licence, neither Angelo nor the government knows if his Newfoundland license has been revoked so he wrote to find out. Angelo still thinks he cannot get his licence till he gets his thesis. Then he is going to apply for an Ontario licence,

After Ottawa, Angelo went to Manpower and Immigration here in Toronto. They had his record since he entered Canada a couple of weeks before. They told him that he could not work as anything but a physician. They also told him there are no immigration charges against him. They told him if there were Federal Immigration charges pending against him, he would never have been allowed back in Canada.

So since Angelo cannot work as a physician till he gets his thesis and cannot work at anything else, he was pretty restless. He wasn't at all happy about the idea of me working and him not. So two weeks ago he left for Finland. That man is difficult to keep up to. You could write half a book on just a month of Angelo's life. Before Angelo left Rome they told him there that Finland really needed doctors. So he checked with the Finnish consulate here and was told the same. So off he went.

He phoned me last week and there were no jobs till October first. So now he is in Italy as far as I know. What his plans are next—that I don't know. He thinks he won't be writing his thesis till the end of November.

Letter from Barbara #2
Friday July 23 1976 Toronto, Ontario

Since I was writing last, I went home for a couple of days and now I'm just getting back to finishing this letter. There was a letter from you to Angelo rerouted from New York to my home, so I sent it on to Italy. I still haven't heard anymore from Angelo---which is rather strange---unless he's mad at me about something---it doesn't take much...

Anyways, Angelo's address in Italy is rather temporary so I won't bother giving it to you. If you are writing to him, I suggest you send it to my home still. That way it can be forwarded to wherever he might be.

I am working at Toronto General Hospital. I was fortunate to get a job since the Nursing situation is very bad here right now. But I had worked there before I went north so I guess that's why. I'm on relief staff which means I still work fulltime but never know what part of the hospital. Most of the time I work in ICU which I like. There are seven ICU's here at TGH so it's interesting and good experience rotating....different from Inuvik General.

My future seems so uncertain. I feel like I am constantly on the move. When Angelo went to Europe I was to follow in a few weeks if he got a job. Now I don't know. We also had set a wedding date October 9 but I think that will be postponed also.

How about your wedding plans? What's everyone saying in Inuvik about Angelo these days? Holli *(nurse friend)* sent me a clipping from The Drum. It was much like the one from the Globe and Mail --- most facts wrong of course.

Well I guess that's all the news for now. Probably Angelo will be writing you and telling you where he's at next. I will be so happy when we are settled down in one place together. I don't care where!

Hope to see you both in the fall.

As ever, Barb

Angelo's Letters
Number 6: from Italy

Dated October 31, 1976
Serracapriola Italy

My dear Lianne,

Barbara sent me your letter and I thank you. I am very happy about your upcoming wedding. May God bless you for all your life. You are my best friends that I will never forget.

Between Barbara and myself it is all over. I will never believe in women again. For all my future life I will continue to love Barbara---she is my only true love. Unfortunately all is over between us. I wish that she will be happy in her life.

On December 2, I will discuss my thesis. The next day I will leave for somewhere in Africa or some other country that will need me to help the poor people.

I want to go far to try to forget Barbara but it is hard. I want to go where I am needed as a doctor without concern for money-

Write to me if you can, it is always nice. Good luck to you and Ron.

I am very unhappy. My intimate life is over. I hope to not live too long because I am suffering so much. Yours truly, Angelo

Angelo's Letters
Number 7: from Rome

Dated November 21, 1976
Rome Italy

Dear Lianne,

I have received the invitation for your wedding. I actually received two of them, one in Serracapriola and another one at my brother's house *(Rome)*. I thank you with all my heart, but it is impossible for me to attend for several reasons. The first one is that on December second, I must write my thesis *(finally)* and right after, I am leaving for a job with the Italian Government, the Minister of the Exterior to help people in third world countries.

It is possible that they will send me to Africa or in South America. They have told me that I must leave by December 10. In any case I thank you very much and wish you a happy life full of love. Alas for me this is not the case but that is life.

Say hello to Ron and tell him that you two are still my best friends for life.

Au revoir,

Love Angelo

Angelo's Letters
Number 8: from Rome

Dated January 30, 1977
Rome Italy

My dear Lianne,

I have received your Christmas letter only a few days ago. I thank you for all your help and I assure you that I will never forget you.

For me life is always the same. I am leaving in a few days for a destination that is unknown to me until forty-eight hours before departure.

I am working overseas in a hospital administered by the Italian government.

If you want you can write to me at this address in Rome.

With all my love as always,

Angelo.

Angelo's Letters
Number 9: from Rome

Dated April 4, 1978
Rome, Italy

Dear Lianne

Only a few days ago I received your nice Christmas card because I have been overseas in Venezuela working for a big company. It was a good work experience especially for tropical diseases. I returned to Rome a week ago but I am ready to return overseas.

I am working for the Italian Government in Sudan Africa where God willing I will be the only doctor for 3,000 people. Italy is building roads there, so the work will take several years. The pay is very low but I must make sacrifices. Well I am content and my medical experiences are increasing.

My private life is as follows. I have not finished my arguments with my ex-wife but the lawyer tells me that in a few months I will have my final divorce.

In December 1976, I met a 29 year old girl who works at Alitalia (*Italian Airline*) and we are together ever since. Now we have a fine son who was born December 6, 1977. His name is Giuseppe DiStefano and I am sending you a picture. We are waiting for my final divorce to get married.

I hope that everything is fine with you. I am glad that you have left Inuvik. If you decide to go on holidays in Italy, remember that my house is always open for you.

Send me some news either at my Rome address or in Sudan.

Love to both of you, Angelo

Angelo's Card
Christmas 1978

Angelo sent me a card from Rome saying:

"My baby on the picture. My wife and I wish you a
Merry Christmas and Happy New Year 1978" from
Angelo and Eliana

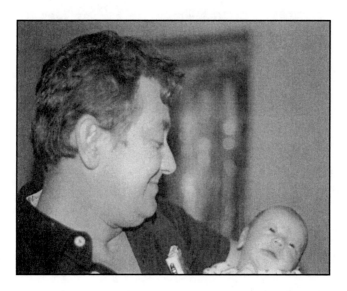

Angelo, finding contentment in his new family.

Angelo's Letters
Number 10: from Venezuela, the last letter

Dated March 3 1981
Caracas, Venezuela
Letterhead says: Dr DiStefano Tarcicio Angelo
Perito Medico Legale Consolato Generale D'Italia

Dear Lianne and Ron

While passing through Rome at the service of the Italian Government I had the pleasure of finding your Christmas card. Thank you. I am very happy to know about your daughter and I am very happy for you all.

For me I am working for a minimum of seven years in Caracas Venezuela. I am in private practice plus I work for the Italian Government doing legal medicine for Italians living here. I travel a lot but I am happy.

As you probably know *(we didn't)* it has been four years since I divorced Stella and I am married to a very intelligent woman called Eliana. We have a son called Giuseppe now three years old.

If you have the time, come and visit us here. There is always sunshine and it is warm all year long. My address is at the bottom of the letter.

As always,

Angelo

Article: "Unmasking Bogus Doctors"

This is an article from a 1982 edition of "Canadian Doctor", a now-defunct medical magazine.

"Is your new colleague really a physician? There's a story of poseurs in the profession and they are not easy to detect...at first."

"The bogus physician has three important con tactics at hand; a winning bedside manner, a ready use of medical jargon and a good or photographic memory. Not only does he develop a rapport with his patients, but he may also gain the respect of his medical colleagues by deferring to their expertise in complicated cases, although this tactic eventually backfires and provides the clue that the good doctor is a con artist."

"And how long an imposter gets away with a scam is directly proportional to the number of practitioners in the area. In a remote community it's easy to pass off yourself off as a doctor for quite a considerable length of time"

"T Angelo Distefano fooled all of the people all of the time in Inuvik N.W.T. for 16 months from 1973 to 1975. As chief surgeon at Inuvik General Hospital, he performed some 360 operations, including successful open heart surgery."

"He left a long trail of fraud, forgery and misrepresentation starting in his native Italy, then in hospitals in Rhodesia and the United States before being granted a provisional licence to practice medicine under the supervision of a qualified physician in Placentia Bay Newfoundland."

"Through a clerical error, his licence became non-provisional, and he moved to Inuvik, an arctic community of 4,000 where he was the only surgeon in the North's largest hospital. Although he was extradited to Italy to face a two year sentence for fraud and forgery, he inspired such confidence in Inuvik that fellow surgeon (*he was the only surgeon remember?*) Dr Ronald Calderisi resigned his position to help Distefano appeal his conviction"

Letter from Lianne Lacroix

Letter to the Editor that was published in September 1982 in "Canadian Doctor"

Dear Sir;

In your article "Unmasking Bogus Doctors" a gross injustice was done to one T. Angelo DiStefano. When a man is accused of a sensational crime by the news media, he is immediately judged and sentenced whether innocent or not.

I spent four years working as G.P. in Inuvik N.W.T. during the time that the alleged impostor was there. I firmly believe his side of the story—that he was a highly trained medical doctor and surgeon whose papers were not in order because of political reasons.

In your article you quote Dr. Carlyle as saying "and how long an impostor gets away with a scam is directly proportional to the number of practitioners in the area". Inuvik is not in the medical boondocks. There were eight G.P.s there over the 16 months working closely with Dr. DiStefano, some with 15 years of experience. Every month we had a specialist from

Edmonton come for a clinic and teaching session. Dr. DiStefano met at least 20 of them.

Every week we had grand rounds going over every patient in the hospital. Dr. DiStefano was an active participant in all of this. We had a lot of bad trauma cases such as stab wounds or gunshot wounds. Dr. DiStefano was always ready and competent. We always assisted in bowel resections or whatever. He told us he had been a resident in Detroit during the racial riots and had performed such surgery there. By his work we agreed that he was obviously well trained.

Your reporter says that he performed successful open heart surgery. This information is incorrect. She also said that he performed some 360 successful operations. That is true! How naive for one to think that an untrained person could possibly perform so many operations with that high rate of success!

For whatever confusion Dr. DiStefano's papers and licences may have become, what makes a doctor is not simply a medical licence that can be gained through fraud, but the years of training. There is no question in our minds that he had the training, the experience plus the dedication to the highest ideals of medicine. This is what makes a doctor – not a piece of paper. After his departure a team of surgeons from Edmonton reviewed over one hundred of his charts. They could find little to criticize.

As for Dr. DiStefano, his problems were political. You see, he is a Communist from his student days in Rome when you can be both a Communist and a Catholic.

For this reason they erased his name from the medical registry in Rome so that he was refused his surgical fellowship in Glasgow on these grounds alone.

I am still in touch with him. He appealed his two year sentence, immediately winning the appeal and his freedom, no doubt because the newly elected Italian government is strongly Communist. At Christmas, he writes to me from Venezuela where he works as an Immigration physician for the Italian government.

Dr. DiStefano: an unusual career yes; an impostor, never!

Yours truly,
L. Lacroix M.D.

Letter from Bill Sara

The Editor- Canadian Doctor
(*now defunct medical magazine*)

October 5, 1982

A letter to the editor from my former colleague Dr L. Lacroix motivated me to seek out your article which I had overlooked, "Unmasking Bogus Doctors". Her criticism of the article is completely legitimate.

After six years of practice in Inuvik, I departed several weeks before Angelo Distefano encountered his difficulties. However my relationship with him up until then, was one of complete professional respect.

I cannot document the 360 operations but my personal records indicate that I provided ninety-six general anesthetics for his surgery including a laparotomy on my wife in which he successfully managed a life threatening problem. Unquestionably I had the utmost confidence in his surgical judgment and technical skill.

As a further testimonial to his credibility and training, let me point out that my own background before Inuvik was a residency in Pathology. Angelo and I were accustomed to reviewing the slides from our surgical and autopsy specimens which were courteously provided by our referral laboratory in Edmonton.

In this regard I feel that I was able to assess him probably more intimately and more objectively than anyone else and I found his academic and histological authority to be entirely satisfactory.

One must reflect critically on this unfair article. There are many other organs to which we may turn to indulge ourselves in poorly researched sensationalism. May the recently announced changes in the editorial personnel of Canadian Doctor correlate with an elevation of journalistic responsibility.

Yours truly,
W. Sara M.D.

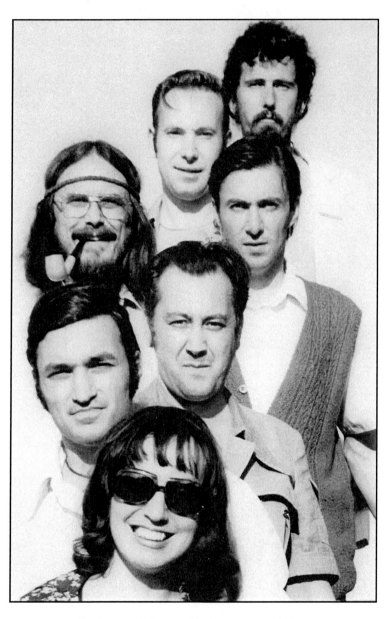

Medical crew of the Inuvik General Hospital, 1975.
Top three: Bill Sara, Rene Tornow (dentist), Stuart McDonald.
Middle three: Frank Kelly, Angelo DiStefano, Ronald Calderisi.
Front: Lianne Lacroix.

Acknowledgments

Writing a book at this time in my life has been a surprise and a delight. I have always enjoyed writing short professional articles and letters to editors of medical journals or local newspapers, but writing a book seemed very far away. Then suddenly a story from my past surfaced, demanding to be told. I was not sure that my writing skills would be up to the task. I wrote a few short chapters and then searched the internet to find an editor who could give me an unbiased opinion.

In this way I found my editor, Jill Veitch, who read my work and liked it! She encouraged my project and has guided my way with helpful suggestions in this new world of writing and publishing a book. For all her help, I am very grateful.

I would also like to thank the Kelowna Library who helped me find a Globe and Mail article from over 30 years ago. They ordered the microfilm from a distant library and thereby gave my story an anchor in history.

This book relates my own unique and wonderful experience in the arctic in the middle 1970's. I was the lone female doctor in a group of keen and lively young doctors. We were learning our profession and enjoying a once in a lifetime experience in the northernmost region of Canada. While the day to day events all blend together in my mind, the medical emergencies and extraordinary moments remain crystal clear. I have changed the names of some people to protect their privacy or because their names have slipped my mind after so many years. In some cases I have combined details from several characters or cases to illustrate a story.

Thank you to my wonderful husband Ron, for his constant encouragement and technical assistance with computers.

Angelo's Fate...

One year after this book was published, Angelo's second cousin, Carl, noticed my website and reached me through the internet. Carl had always wondered about Angelo, mentioning that the surgeon had been a figure of mystery even to his own relatives. Carl remembered him from the 1976 visit where Angelo and Barbara had stayed at his family's house in New York. Carl had lost track of him over the years but had recently learned of Angelo's death in 2009. Through various aunts and cousins the rest of the story was pieced together. It would appear that Angelo's relationship with Eliana ended early in 1981 and they never legally married. She returned to Italy with their son, Guiseppe, who is not in contact with the rest of the family.

Later that same year Angelo met and married Rosita and they settled in San Cristobal, Venezuela. Rosita herself has emailed me further details of their life. At the time of his death, Angelo was the founder and medical director of a surgical clinic that employed over a dozen medical specialists and numerous staff. It was more like a small hospital with full diagnostic services, an obstetric department and pediatrics, and even cancer treatment. Angelo never retired and was still working as a general surgeon until he became ill and died of renal failure at age 74. Angelo and Rosita are the proud parents of two daughters, Rosangela and Karina, young adults in their mid-20s, who are university students in dentistry and medicine.

It pleases me greatly to know that Angelo spent the last three decades of his life enjoying a lovely family and helping people by doing what he loved the best—surgery. He was obviously highly regarded by his peers and cherished by his family.

In the end that is all we can ask of life...   LL

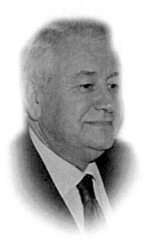

Dr. Angelo Tarcisio Centuori di Stefano
July 13, 1935 — April 14, 2009

On April 14, 2009 Dr. Angelo Di Stefano, surgeon and founder of the San Sebastian Surgical Clinic left us on this earth.

Even absent he will continue to make his mark in the task of serving others with perseverance, dedication and determination as he did always.

He touched the lives of many and we pay tribute to his memory that will forever live in our hearts.*

*translation